PEDIATRIC OBSTRUCTIVE SLEEP APNEA

DR.B.SUBHA

notionpress.com

INDIA • SINGAPORE • MALAYSIA

ISBN

Paperback 979-8-90451-012-1
Hardcase 979-8-90451-013-8

Contents

Acknowledgement

I express my heartfelt gratitude on the publication of my book ***Obstructive Sleep Apnea****. This work would not have been possible without the constant support, encouragement, and guidance of many people who stood by me throughout this journey.*

The publication of this book marks not only an academic milestone but also a deeply personal journey. I am incredibly grateful to my parents, ***Mr. R. Babu Ashok*** *and* ***Mrs. M. Karthikeyini****, whose unwavering love, selflessness, and unceasing support have molded me into the person I am today. My biggest base has always been their unshakable faith in my skills.Every achievement of mine is a reflection of their values, guidance, and blessings.*

I extend my heartfelt thanks to my dear brother, ***Mr. B. Vaseekar****, for his continued support, motivation, and confidence in me. His encouragement has always inspired me to strive for excellence.*

My special and sincere appreciation goes to my husband, ***Dr. I. Kathiravan****, Endodontist whose patience, understanding, and steadfast support have been my pillar of strength throughout this journey. His emotional support and encouragement during the demanding phases of writing and compiling this book have been invaluable.*

I am profoundly grateful to my respected staff members — ***Dr. Rena Ephraim, Dr. Ambili Ayiliath, Dr. Sharath Chandrashekar, Dr. Dhanya K.B., Dr. Mridhul, Dr. Ramnesh, and Dr. Fazila*** *— for their professional cooperation, constructive suggestions, and continuous encouragement. Their support has contributed significantly to the successful completion of this publication.*

I also acknowledge all my teachers, mentors, and well-wishers who have directly or indirectly contributed to my academic growth and inspired me to undertake this work. Each interaction, discussion, and shared experience has enriched this book in meaningful ways.

Finally, I extend my gratitude to everyone who supported me behind the scenes and encouraged me to bring this vision into reality. May this book serve as a valuable resource and contribute meaningfully to the understanding and management of obstructive sleep apnea.

Last but not the least, I thank the ***ALMIGHTY GOD*** *for his blessings and providing me strength, courage and perseverance to make my vision a reality.*

With sincere gratitude,

Dr. B. Subha

ABBREVIATION	FULL FORM
SRBD	Sleep Related Breathing Disorders
OSA	Obstructive sleep apnea
SDB	Sleep Disordered Breathing
CA	Central Apnea
PSG	Polysomnography
REM	Rapid Eye Movement
NREM	Non -Rapid Eye Movement
OHS	Obesity Hypoventilation Syndrome
AASM	American Academy of Sleep Medicine
ECG	Electrocardiogram
RDI	Respiratory Disturbance Index
EEG	Electroencephalogram
PLMD	Periodic Limb Movement Disorder
UA anatomy	Upper airway anatomy
SEPAR	Spanish Society of Pneumology and Thoracic Surgery
AHI	Apnea- hypopnea index
CPAP	Continuous Positive Airway Pressure
QoL	Quality Of Life index
NPPV	Non-invasive Positive Pressure Ventilation
RME	Rapid Maxillary Expansion
OSAHS	obstructive sleep apnea hypopnoea syndrome
FTP	Friedman tongue Position
CBC	Complete Blood Count
CVS	Cardiovascular system

CNS	Central Nervous System
TSH	Thyroid Stimulating Hormone
ICSD	International Classification of Sleep Disorders
OCST	out-of-center sleep testing
RERAs	Respiratory effort related arousals
REI	Respiratory Event Index
ESS	Epworth Sleepiness Scale
HSAT	Home Sleep Apnea Test
CVA	Cerebrovascular Accident
CHF	Chronic heart failure
PH	Pulmonary Hypertension
NAFLD	Non-alcoholic fatty liver disease
CHAT	Childhood Adenotonsillectomy Trial
AAP	American Academy of Pediatrics
DISE	Drug induced sleep endoscopy
MAD	Mandibular Advancement Device
TSD	Tongue stabilizing Device
MMA	Maxillomandibular advancement

Introduction

It is believed that sleep is crucial to a child's healthy development. Breathing abnormalities during sleep have the potential to interfere with sleep in addition to their effect on gas exchange. The four subgroups of sleep-related breathing disorders (SRBDs) under the international classification of sleep disorders include central sleep apnea, obstructive sleep apnea (OSA), sleep-related hypoventilation disorders, and sleep-related hypoxemia disorder.

A broad spectrum of abnormalities in gas exchange, respiratory rhythm, and sleep architecture are together referred to as "sleep disordered breathing" (SDB). 2 SDB is made up of:

Obstructive sleep apnea (OSA), which is characterized by episodes of complete or partial airway blockage; central apnea (CA), which is characterized by prolonged pauses without respiratory effort; and hypoventilation, which is characterized by persistent low tidal volume breathing or bradypnea that causes hypercarbia and hypoxemia. 3 The most common subtype of SDB, OSA, affects 15% of children in good health. 4 The most frequent cause of OSA in children in good health is adenotonsillar hypertrophy. Adenotonsillectomy (AT) is the first treatment for OSA.

In children, OSA is defined as a respiratory condition that causes partial or complete upper airway obstruction when they sleep, which hinders breathing and interferes with sleep. It is a disorder when the back of the throat muscles sporadically relax excessively, obstructing the airway either entirely or partially. This indicates that the infant may be breathing intermittently while they are asleep. These breathing pauses might occur five to more than thirty times in an hour, and they usually last ten to twenty seconds.

OSA is described by the American Thoracic Society as a "functional disturbance in sleep characterized by transient and partial/complete obstruction of the airways which interrupts sleep, resulting in disruption of normal gas exchange (intermittent hypoxia and hypercapnia) and sleep fragmentation."" 2 The first systematic description of OSA in children was conducted in 1976 using polysomnography (PSG) and clinical symptoms.[3]

Since then, the identification of irregular breathing during sleep has advanced significantly during the past 20 years, and it has become clear that childhood OSA is both prevalent and dangerous.

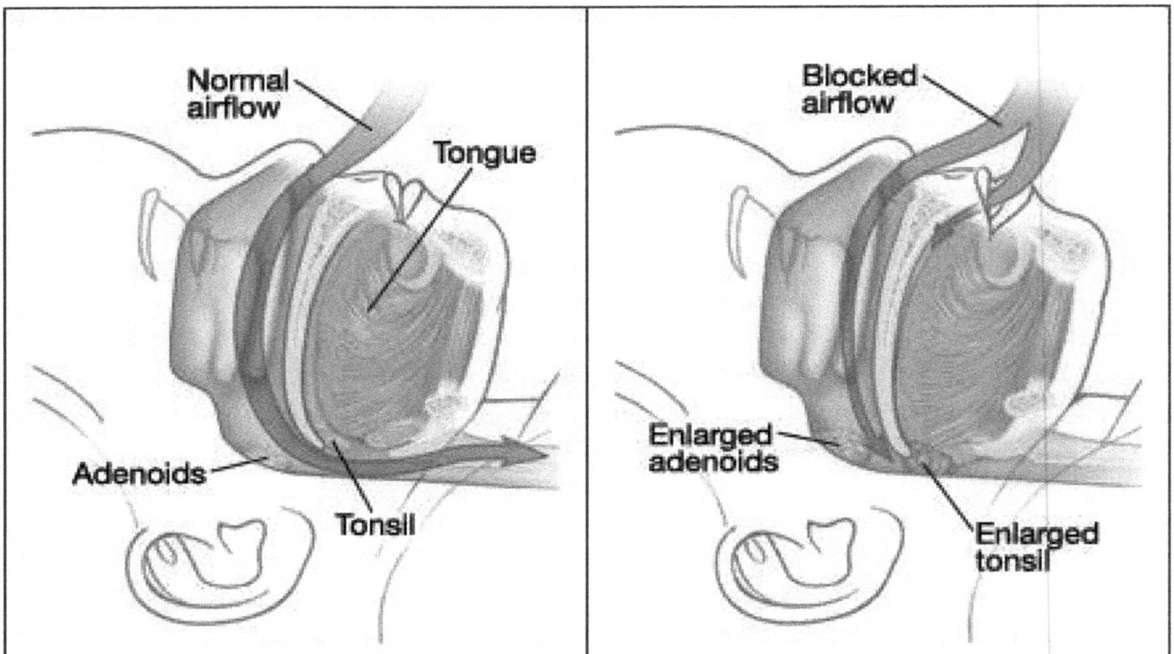

Air normally flows freely from the nose to the lungs.	When your child has OSA, airflow through the throat is blocked during sleep.
Normal airflow	Obstructive sleep apnea

Although there is still more to learn, our understanding of the pathophysiology has increased. The connection between respiratory irregularities during sleep and negative outcomes is becoming better acknowledged.

When they sleep, children with OSA typically breathe differently than adults. Compared to adults, children have a higher threshold for arousal. 4 Because of this, they often do not awaken in reaction to obstructive events, and the majority of research has shown that sleep architecture is either preserved or just slightly altered. In contrast, OSA in adulthood is linked to reduced slow wave and rapid eye movement (REM) sleep as well as severe sleep fragmentation (6,7,8). Due to relative muscle atonia, a state-specific impairment in upper airway function, OSA is typically more severe in children during REM sleep.

The syndrome is more prevalent in older and middle-aged people. The complex process of upper airway collapse, which includes pharyngeal neuropathy, fluid shift towards the neck, obesity, craniofacial abnormalities, and altered upper airway muscle function, is unknown. The collapse's primary consequences include intermittent hypoxia and hypercapnia, frequent arousals, increased respiratory effort, secondary sympathetic activation, oxidative stress, and systemic inflammation.

Cardiovascular comorbidities such as hypertension, arrhythmias, stroke, coronary heart disease, atherosclerosis, overall elevated cardiovascular mortality, and metabolic dysfunction are also linked to obstructive sleep apnea syndrome (OSAS). Carefully structured research has yet to determine if treating sleep apnea can completely eradicate its long-term effects.

Obesity hypoventilation syndrome (OHS) was first characterized by Bickelmann et al. 9 in a 1956 report on an obese company boss who arrived at the hospital complaining of excessive daily sleepiness. Because of the way a comparable fictional character was described in Charles Dickens' first novel (1836–1837), these experts named the disease Pickwickian syndrome. Posthumous records of the Pickwick Club. Under the umbrella of sleep-disordered breathing (SDB), other descriptions of obese hypoventilation syndrome, obstructive sleep apnea, and central sleep apnea were later published.

Currently, obstructive sleep apnea (OSA) is the most prevalent and clinically significant SDB. Heart failure, atrial fibrillation, pulmonary hypertension, hypertension, and cerebrovascular accidents are among the conditions it has been associated with.[10]

SLEEP

Cardiovascular, cerebrovascular, and metabolic health, as well as mood, mental health, and cognitive performance, all depend on getting enough sleep. 11 Untreated sleep disorders, circadian misalignment, short-term sleep deprivation, and long-term sleep restriction can all have significant negative effects on one's physical, mental, and emotional well-being as well as public safety. Chronic sleep deprivation raises the chance of death and increases the personal and societal burden of a number of disease conditions epidemics, including heart disease, diabetes, cancer, and obesity. 12 Both self-rating and objective sleep continuity criteria can demonstrate the qualities of healthy sleep, which include adequate duration, appropriate time, regularity, the absence of sleep problems, and acceptable quality.13, 14

POLYSOMNOGRAPHY

A sleep study, or polysomnography, is an electrophysiological research that uses simultaneous multiparameter recordings to measure oxygenation, awakening events, apneahypopnea episodes, and the quality of sleep. In order to investigate sleep disorders, the American Academy of Sleep Medicine (AASM) scoring guideline suggests using a combination of electroencephalogram, electromyogram, electrooculogram, ECG, oronasal airflow, end-tidal CO2, and oxygen saturation (SpO2). The data measured during a sleep study are used to calculate the apnea-hypopnea index (AHI), respiratory disturbance index (RDI), and degree of hypoventilation. When doing a sleep study, it's critical to recognize the differences between adults and children.

Physiology of Sleep

The fundamental structural arrangement of regular sleep is known as sleep architecture. Rapid eye movement (REM) and non-REM sleep are the two types of sleep. A range of relative depth is reflected in the NREM sleep stages 1, 2, 3, and 4. Each has distinct traits, such as differences in muscle tone, eye movements, and brain wave patterns. Electroencephalographic (EEG) recordings, which track the electrical patterns of brain activity, were used to identify sleep cycles and stages. 15. During a sleep period, REM and NREM sleep alternate cyclically (Fig 1). Sleep disorders are linked to irregular cycling and/or absent sleep stages, while the purpose of the alternations between these two types of sleep is yet unknown. 16. For instance, people with narcolepsy go straight into REM sleep rather than the usual NREM sleep.

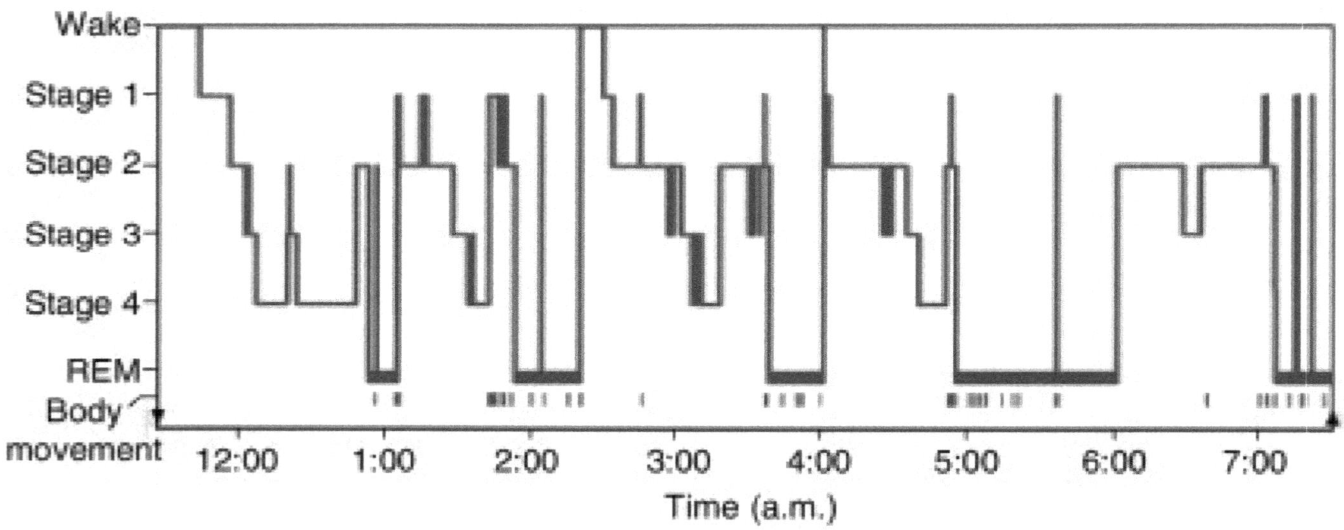

Fig 1: Showing Progression of sleep states across a single night in young adult.

Sleep Cycles: NREM and REM

A brief interval of NREM stage 1 precedes stages 2, 3, and 4, and finally REM during a sleep episode. Nevertheless, people alternate between NREM and REM sleep stages during the night rather than being in REM sleep for the entire duration (Fig 1).

Between 75 and 80 percent of sleep is NREM, with the remaining 20 to 25 percent being REM. The initial NREM-REM sleep cycle typically lasts between 70 and 100 minutes. The second and subsequent cycles last between ninety and one hundred and twenty minutes. REM sleep lengthens in the latter portion of a sleep episode and rises throughout the night in most persons. Stage 2 starts to make up the majority of NREM sleep as the sleep episode goes on, and stages 3 & 4 may occasionally completely vanish.

Four Stages of NREM Sleep

Each of the four phases of NREM sleep is linked to distinct physiology and brain activity. The usual EEG patterns for each of the four NREM stages are depicted in the graphic below.

To monitor discernible changes in muscle tone and eye movement, additional tools are utilized.

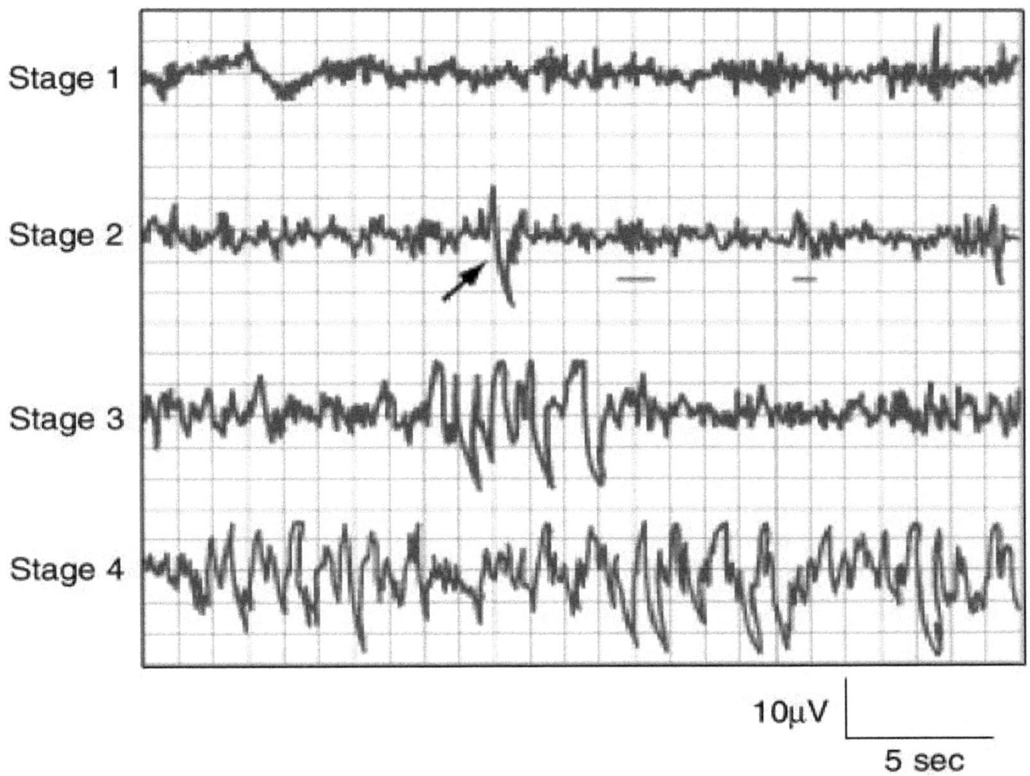

Fig 2: Showing EEG activity Characteristics for four stages of NREM sleep.

NOTE: a K-complex is indicated by the arrow in stage two, and two sleep spindles are indicated by the underlining.

REM Sleep

Muscle atonia, bursts of fast eye movements, and desynchronized (low-voltage, mixed-frequency) brain wave activities are characteristics of REM sleep. REM sleep is also characterized by slow alpha activity, sawtooth wave patterns, and theta activity (3 to 7 counts per second). The REM phase may only last one to five minutes during the first cycle, but it gets longer as the sleep episode goes on. 18. NREM and REM sleep differ in several physiological ways.

Physiological Process	NREM	REM

Brain activity	Decreases from wakefulness	Increases in motor and sensory areas, while other areas are similar to NREM
Heart rate	Slows from wakefulness	Increases and varies compared to NREM
Blood pressure	Decreases from wakefulness	Increases (up to 30 percent) and varies from NREM
Sympathetic nerve activity	Decreases from wakefulness	Increases significantly from wakefulness
Muscle tone	Similar to wakefulness	Absent
Blood flow to brain	Decreases from wakefulness	Increases from NREM, depending on brain region
Respiration	Decreases from wakefulness	Increases and varies from NREM, but may show brief stoppages; coughing suppressed
Airway resistance	Increases from wakefulness	Increases and varies from wakefulness
Body temperature	Is regulated at lower set point than wakefulness; shivering initiated at lower temperature than During wakefulness	Is not regulated; no shivering or sweating; temperature drifts toward that of the local environment
Sexual arousal	Occurs infrequently	Greater than NREM

Table 1: Comparison of NREM and REM sleep [19]

REM sleep is most frequently linked to dreaming. Loss of reflexes and muscle tone probably has a significant purpose since it keeps a person from acting out their nightmares or dreams while they're asleep.

SLEEP-WAKE REGULATION

The Two-Process Model

It is believed that two main systems interact to control the sleep-wake system: process S, which promotes sleep, and process C, which keeps one awake. 18. Process S is the homeostatic need for sleep. Process S, or the urge for sleep, increases throughout the day, peaks just before bed, and then decreases at night.

The circadian system controls Process C, which promotes wakefulness. Throughout the day, process C develops to oppose process S and encourage attentiveness and wakefulness. But as the urge for sleep wanes throughout the night, this wake-promoting system starts to diminish at bedtime, improving sleep consolidation. 19. After getting a good night's sleep, the circadian waking drive starts to raise, the homeostatic desire for sleep decreases, and the cycle restarts. Because total sleep time is consistent but distributed randomly throughout the day and night in the absence of process C, process C also serves to combine waking and sleep into somewhat distinct episodes.[19]

Importantly, mechanism C synchronizes the circadian clock to keep sleep-wakefulness cycles in line with environmental light-dark cycles.

CIRCADIAN RHYTHMS, THE 24-HOUR CLOCK

Circadian rhythms are the collective term for the daily cycles in behavior and physiology. Throughout the day, they regulate body temperature, heart rate, muscle tone, hormone secretion, and the sleep-wake cycle. They also regulate food intake and physical activity. Neural structures in the hypothalamus that serve as a biological clock produce the rhythms.19. Endogenous clocks are used by both plants and animals to coordinate daily physiological and behavioral cycles with the external day-night cycle. Twenty A number of biochemical pathways including clock genes that are expressed in a roughly 24-hour rhythm are thought to constitute the foundation for these clocks.

In mammals, two proteins known as Clock and Bmal1 unite and travel to the nucleus of the cell, where they bind to certain DNA sequences that trigger particular genes (Fig. 3). They activate several genes, including Cryptochrome and Period. Furthermore, these genes' products return to the nucleus, where they prevent Clock and Bmal1 from being produced by interfering with their capacity to bind to DNA. Because of this, the products of the Period and Cryptochrome genes show a rising and falling pattern of expression having a very nearly 24-hour periodicity.

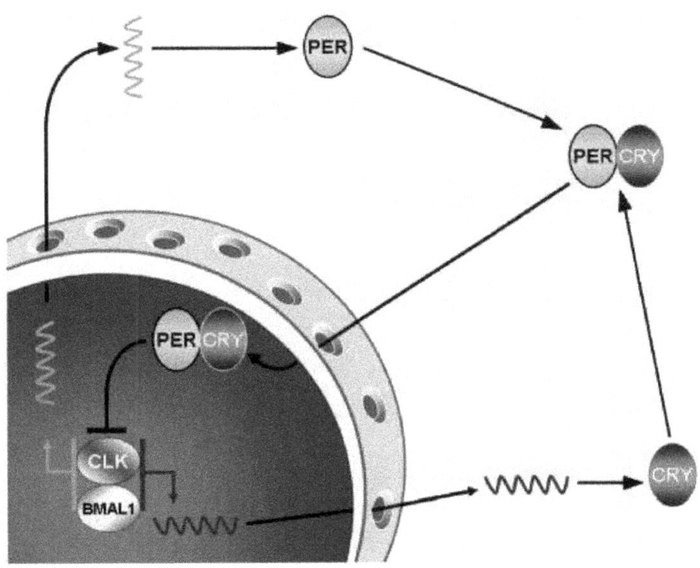

Fig:3 Showing Molecular mechanisms that underpin the action of the circadian clock.

NOTE : Circadian clocks' 24-hour cycle time is controlled by a negative feedback loop that involves the activation and deactivation of Period and Cryptochrome proteins. As a result, the Period and Cryptochrome proteins' ability to modify their own production enables the system to regulate itself.

Numerous other genes that cycle in various bodily tissues and produce daily activity patterns are likewise regulated by clock and Bmal1. The circadian system is involved in many aspects of life, as evidenced by the numerous cellular processes that these rhythmically expressed genes support, such as oxidative metabolism, secretion, signal transduction, glucose and lipid metabolism, and many more.

SLEEP DISORDERS BREATHING

Sleep disordered breathing (SDB) is a comprehensive term that refers to irregularities in respiratory patterns, gas exchange, and sleep architecture during sleep. Sleep disorders refer to a wide range of diseases that have serious effects for individual health and huge societal expenses. Categorization of sleep disorders Pharmacological and nonpharmacological therapy methods are evaluated, and primary and secondary insomnia are differentiated. Treatments like chronotherapy and light therapy are described in conjunction with common circadian rhythm issues.

There is discussion of the diagnosis and treatment of periodic limb movement disorder and restless legs syndrome. Treatments for upper airway resistance syndrome and obstructive sleep apnea are the primary subjects of discussion. Along with diagnostic tests and treatment, the constellation of symptoms and findings associated with narcolepsy is examined. Sleep terrors, somnambulism, and rapid eye movement (REM) behavior sleep disorders are examples of parasomnias that are detailed, along with the outcomes of laboratory tests and available treatments.

Classification of sleep disorders

Sleep disorders fall into four main groups according to the International Classification of Sleep Disorders diagnostic and coding manual from 2000: sleep disorders, parasomnias, and dyssomnias.

Dyssomnias	Parasomnias	Sleep disorders associated with mental, neurological, or other medical disorders	Proposed sleep disorders
Intrinsic sleep disorders	Arousal disorders	Associated with mental disorders	Short sleeper
Psycho physiological insomnia	Confusional arousals	Psychoses	Long sleeper
Sleep state misperceptio	Sleepwalking	Mood disorders	Sub wakefulnes syndrome
Idiopathic insomnia	Sleep terrors	Anxiety disorder	Fragmentary myoclonus
Narcolepsy	Sleep-wake transition disorder	Panic disorders	Sleep hyperhidrosis
Recurrent hypersomnia	Rhythmic starts	Alcoholism	Menstrual associated sleep disorder
Idiopathic hypersomnia	Sleep starts	Associated with neurological disorder	Pregnancy associated sleep disorder

Post traumatic hypersomnia	Sleep talking	Cerebral degenerative disorders	Terrifying hypnagogic hallucinations
Central alveolar hypo-ventilation syndrome	Nocturnal leg cramps	Dementia	Sleep-related neurogenic tachypnea
Periodic limb movemen disorder	Parasomnias usually associated with REM sleep	Parkinsonism	Sleep-related laryngospasm

Table 2: Showing Classification of Sleeping Disorders [8]

Dyssomnias symptoms include extreme sleepiness and trouble falling or staying asleep. 5. Sleep disorders can be classified as intrinsic, extrinsic, or circadian rhythm based on their pathophysiological processes. 5 Intrinsic sleep disorders are problems that originate or arise within the body. Narcolepsy, obstructive sleep apnea syndrome, restless legs syndrome, idiopathic and psychophysiological insomnia, and periodic limb movement disorder (PLMD) are examples of common intrinsic sleep disorders.

4 Unwanted behavioral & physical changes, mainly during sleep, are the hallmark of parasomnias. 5 They include sleep-stage transitions, partial arousal, and arousal issues.

Mental illnesses like alcoholism, schizophrenia, mood disorders, anxiety disorders, and panic disorders are also associated with sleep problems. Neurological conditions such as brain degenerative disorders, dementia, parkinsonism, fatal familial insomnia, sleep-related epilepsy, sleep-induced electrical status epilepticus, and migraines are linked to sleep problems.

Among the proposed sleep disorders are subwakefulness syndrome, fragmented myoclonus, menstrual-associated sleep disorder, pregnancy-associated sleep disorder, horrifying hypnagogic hallucinations, sleep-related neurogenic tachypnea, sleep-related laryngospasm, and sleep choking syndrome.5

Sleep disorders are a common category of ailments that have negative effects on people's health and cost society money. The diagnosis of sleep disorders requires careful history taking, physical examination, and laboratory testing. Even while there are general recommendations for treating the more prevalent and severe sleep disorders, each patient's treatment must be customized.

Obstructive Sleep Apnea

Episodes of complete (apnea) or partial collapse (hypopnea) of the upper airway combined with a decrease in oxygen saturation or waking from sleep are the hallmarks of obstructive sleep apnea (OSA). 22 Sleep is fragmented and non-restorative as a result of this disturbance. Additional symptoms include increased daytime fatigue, loud, bothersome snoring, and confirmed apneas during sleep. OSA has a major impact on quality of life, mental health, cardiovascular health, and driving safety.24

Etiology

Numerous factors contribute to the complex phenomenon of pharyngeal narrowing and closure during sleep. Upper airway obstruction during sleep is anticipated to be significantly influenced by anatomic risk factors, neuromuscular characteristics, and sleep-induced decreased ventilatory drive. 22 Anatomical components that contribute to pharyngeal narrowing include large neck circumference, soft tissue, bone, and arteries. Increased pressure surrounding the upper airway can be caused by many of these structures, which can result in pharyngeal collapse and insufficient space for airflow to a portion of the upper airway during sleep.25 25. Additionally, the tone of the upper airway muscles is important; a recurrent whole or partial airway collapse happens when this muscle deteriorates. The main causes of OSA in adults are obesity, male sex, and aging. 26. After controlling for body mass index, the severity of OSA diminishes with age.27

Anatomical factors

- Micrognathia and retrognathia
- The elongation of the face
- Mandibular hypoplasia
- Tonsillar and adenoid hypertrophy
- The hyoid's inferior displacement

Non-anatomic Risk Factors

- The distribution of central fat
- Obesity
- Advanced age
- Gender: male
- Sleeping in a supine position

- Being pregnant

Additional factors

- Drinking alcohol
- The act of smoking
- The application of hypnotics and sedatives

Associated Medical Disorders

- Endocrine conditions, such as hypothyroidism, metabolic syndrome, diabetes mellitus, and acromegaly
- Neurological conditions, such as myasthenia gravis, stroke, and spinal cord injuries
- Prader Willi syndrome
- Down syndrome
- Heart failure that is congestive
- Fibrillation of the atrium
- Hypoventilation syndrome associated with obesity

FOUR PHENOTYPES OF OBSTRUCTIVE SLEEP APNEA

The OSA phenotype can be operationally defined as:

Patients with OSA are classified based on clinically relevant factors such as symptoms, treatment response, health consequences, and quality of life.

Aim of Phenotyping: -

- Enhancing comprehension of disease mechanisms
- Anticipating treatment reaction
- Danger of unfavorable outcomes
- Reducing clinical trial heterogeneity

Ideally, the phenotype reflects an endotype, which is a subtype of disease with a consistent natural history, clinical and physiological characteristics, identifiable pathobiology, and predictable response to therapies affecting patient outcomes.28

Phenotypes without all the characteristics of an endotype may become closer to that status as supporting data (genetics, genomes, and biologic markers) are acquired. Prognosis and treatment may become even more precise as a result of this enhancement. Because certain traits, including excessive daytime sleepiness, fragmented sleep, or treatment-resistant hypertension, may be considered outcomes or phenotypes, the outcomes used in phenotypic identification should be well defined.

Phenotyping Approaches

Phenotyping techniques can be categorized according to their characteristics (clinical vs molecular, for example) and experimental strategies (supervised versus unsupervised). Establishing discrete patient categories based on signs like indications, symptoms, demographics, comorbidities, physiological and anatomical measures, or therapy responsiveness is the focus of clinical phenotyping 29. Using molecular traits including DNA, RNA, mRNA, miRNA, proteins, metabolites, and other biological products, molecular phenotyping aims to identify individuals. Additionally, the approach may incorporate thousands of features (single nucleotide polymorphisms) or just one (sex).

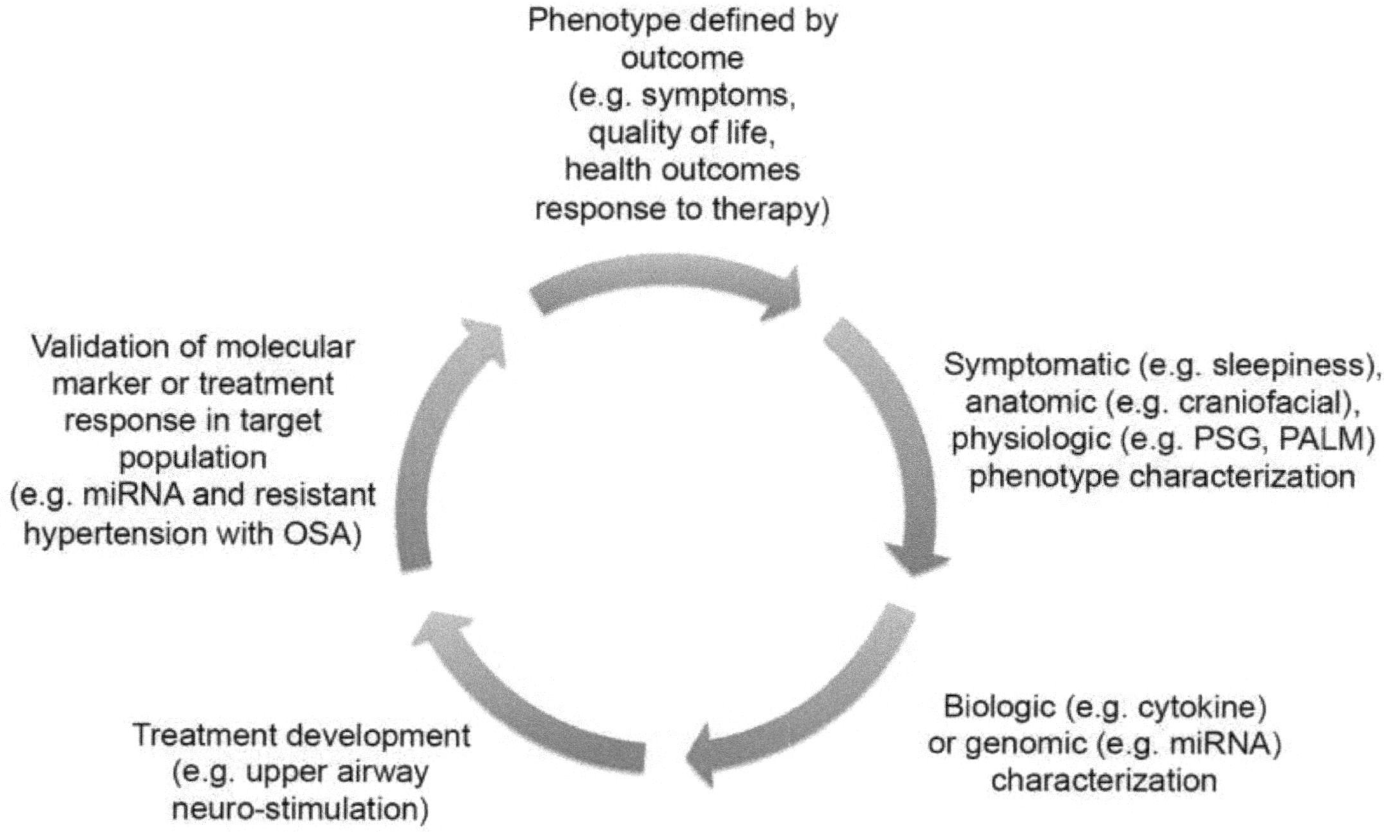

Fig 4 Showing Alterative process of phenotype identification and validation in obstructive sleep apnea (OSA)

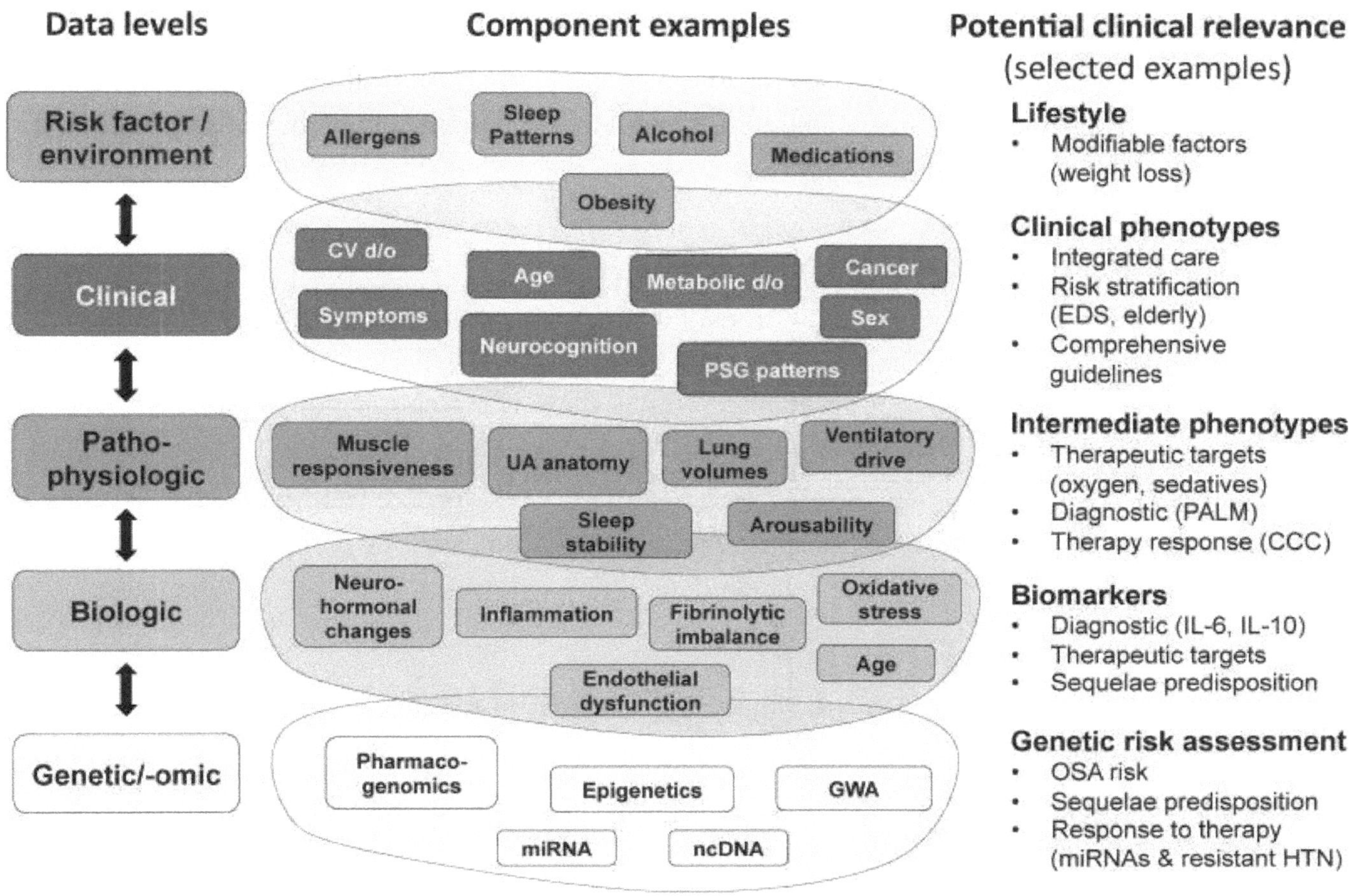

Fig 5 Showing Data levels in obstructive sleep apnea (OSA) phenotyping and the potential benefits

DIAGNOSIS OF OBSTRUCTIVE SLEEP APNEA

A comprehensive history, a clinical examination, and, finally, an endoscopic and instrumental assessment comprise the clinical evaluation of a juvenile OSA patient. According to reports, the clinical examination and history have a positive predictive value of 46% and 65%, respectively, for the diagnosis of OSA. However, when choosing patients for instrumental testing such as PSG, clinical evaluation is helpful. The Spanish 30, European 31, and American 32 guidelines explain the clinical recommendations that determine the diagnosis of OSA in the pediatric population.

To increase diagnostic efficiency, this manual separates the OSA diagnostic method into main care and inpatient treatment.

A medical history and a comprehensive clinical examination should be performed in primary care for children with suspected OSA (snoring, symptoms, or suggestive clinical findings).

1. Medical history includes family history, sleep and breathing events, and the Chervin sleep questionnaire.
2. Conduct a comprehensive clinical examination, including craniofacial and UA anatomy, cardiovascular assessment, and somatometry. Obese children are a particularly vulnerable demographic. Depending on the results, the patient may be referred from primary care to a reference sleep facility.

Spanish Society of Pneumology and Thoracic Surgery (SEPAR)

1. Hospital RP is conducted if OSA is suspected based on clinical history, including Chervin, retrognathia, adenotonsillar hypertrophy, and Mallampati score > 2. Otherwise, a control visit is conducted six months after the baseline visit.
2. Adenotonsillar surgery is recommended for children with a respiratory event index of 5 or above in the RP. When the results are poor, a PSG is used.
3. For PSG patients with an AHI ≥ 5/h, adenotonsillar surgery is advised. Anti-inflammatory medication or a 6-month review visit are advised if the AHI is less than 3/h. For an AHI of three to five hours, comorbidities are evaluated. Adenotonsillectomy is done when comorbidity is present, and anti-inflammatory drugs are utilized when it is not.
4. Children with severe preoperative OSA or persistent symptoms should undergo a clinical reassessment within 6 months of surgery. Treatment options such as diet, CPAP, or orthodontics may be considered.

European Respiratory Society

1. Identifying risk factors for SDB, including UA obstruction symptoms, physical exam changes, objective findings, preterm, and family history.
2. Identify any disorders that coexist with SDB, such as nocturnal enuresis, metabolic syndrome, wheeze or asthma, tympanostomy tube implantation, oral-motor dysfunction, and recurrent otitis media.
3. Identifying the risk variables for long-term SDB, including African-American race, obesity, male sex, obstructive AHI > 5/h, small mandibles, and persistent tonsillar hypertrophy.
4. Objective diagnosis and severity evaluation of SDB: For children at risk of SDB, PSG or RP is advised. (1) OSA definition 1: obstructive apnea index ≥ 1/h or obstructive AHI ≥ 2/h with symptoms of SDB; (2) OSA definition 2: SDB symptoms plus AHI ≥ 1/h. Although there are no PSG substitutes, the Pediatric Sleep Questionnaire, the Sleep Clinical Record, ambulatory PSG or RP, and nocturnal oximetry could be used in low-resource situations.
5. When AHI is more than five per hour, SDB treatment is advised. In the absence of PSG or RP, therapy is recommended if there is positive oximetry, SDB questionnaires, or morbidity. Whether main snoring should be treated (annual evaluation) is debatable.
6. To fully resolve SDB, a step-by-step therapeutic approach is usually employed. (1) Children who are overweight or obese may lose weight.For children under the age of six who are not obese, treatment options for OSA include nasal corticosteroids and/or montelukast; craniofacial surgery for syndromic craniofacial abnormalities; tracheostomy for severe OSA; rapid maxillary expansion or orthodontic app liances for children with maxillary constriction, retrognathia, or malocclusion; and adenotonsillectomy for children with adenotonsillar hypertrophy.
7. Monitoring symptoms, PSG, QoL, CV/CNS morbidity, enuresis, and growth rate following treatments are all part of managing persistent SDB. Children with persistent symptoms, children at risk of developing chronic OSA after adenotonsillectomy, and children with mild OSA receiving

corticosteroids and/or montelukast should have PSG or RP six to twelve weeks after treatment. PSG should be carried out six months after choosing to use an oral appliance and twelve months after rapid maxillary expansion. CPAP or NPPV should be titrated using at least one PSG or RP annually.

American Academy of Paediatrics

1. OSA screening. Doctors should perform a physical examination and medical history if the child has symptoms or indicators of OSA.
2. Snoring should be evaluated using PSG (the gold standard test) or other techniques (such as nighttime video recording, nocturnal oximetry, daytime nap PSG, or ambulatory PSG).
3. Unless surgery is contraindicated, adenotonsillectomy is recommended for children with OSA and adenotonsillar hypertrophy. Other therapies should be pursued if the child has OSA but no adenotonsillar hypertrophy.
4. Adenotonsillectomy patients at high risk are monitored.
5. Rethink. whether symptoms continue after therapy, all OSA patients should have a clinical assessment to see whether further treatment is necessary (6 to 8 weeks after treatment).
6. If symptoms persist after adenotonsillectomy or if surgery is not done, refer patients for CPAP treatment.
7. If a child with OSA is overweight or obese, weight loss should be combined with other therapies
8. Children with mild OSA who are unable to have surgery or who have mild postoperative OSA (<5/h) may benefit from intranasal corticosteroids.

TYPES OF PEDIATRIC OBSTRUCTIVE SLEEP APNEA

Two forms of OSA in children have been identified based on adenotonsillar hypertrophy and elevated fat deposits in upper airway tissues.33

In the absence of obesity, Type I is linked to substantial lymphadenoid enlargement. Type II is primarily associated with moderate upper airway lymphadenoid hyperplasia and obesity.

Symptoms and Findings similar in OSA Type I and Type II [33]

- Regular snoring (at least three nights a week)
- Frequent awakenings during agitated sleep
- The diaphoresis
- Nightmares and terrors at night
- Wetting in bed
- Parents reported breathing pauses.
- Stuffy nose and nasal speaking pattern
- Restricted nasal airflow and mouth breathing
- Frequent trips to the primary care physician for problems connected to the respiratory system

- The retrognathia

S.NO	Characteristic feature	OSA TYPE I	OSA TYPE II
1.	Excessive daytime sleepiness	+	++++
2.	Weight gain	-	++
3.	Hyperactive behavior	++++	- Or +
4.	Attention problems	++++	+++
5.	Truncal/visceral obesity	-or +	+++
6.	Enlarged neck circumference	– or +	+++
7.	Enlarged tonsils/adenoids	++++	++
8.	Recurrent otitis media/tympanostomy tube placement	+++	+
9.	Depression and low self-esteem	+	+++
10.	Shyness and social withdrawal	+	+++
11.	Left ventricular hypertrophy	++	++++

12.	Systemic hypertension/altered blood pressure regulation	+	++++
13.	Insulin resistance	-	++++
14.	Serum lipid abnormalities	+	++++
15.	Elevated C-reactive protein	++	++++
16.	Elevated liver enzymes	-	++

Table 4 showing Symptoms and Findings Relatively Specific to OSA Types I and II

An additional pediatric category in the nomenclature of OSA (i.e., type III) addressed some of the unique presentation and outcome characteristics of children with a variety of craniofacial and neuromuscular disorders (such as Crouzon and Apert syndromes, Pierre Robin sequence, Down syndrome, Goldenhar syndrome, achondroplasia, myelomeningocele, and cerebral palsy).33

CHARACTERISTICS OF OBSTRUCTIVE SLEEP APNEA

Weight

People with OSA who are overweight or obese make up two thirds. Whether the person has always been overweight or if the weight gain happened recently is irrelevant. Another common feature of OSA is a wide neck circumference (a collar size larger than 17 inches for men), which is frequently suggestive of fatty tissue surrounding the airway.

In certain research, OSA was more strongly predicted by neck size than by the degree of obesity.

Head & Face

OSA is associated with certain aspects of the head and face. A short lower jaw (mandible), where the chin is clearly behind the upper jaw and does not extend behind it, is one that can be seen with a simple external examination. This is often referred to as retrognathia. Additional findings that require in-depth investigation or specialist research include:

- A big tongue
- The little airway behind the tongue
- The tonsils are large.
- A thicker, longer soft palate
- The hyoid bone's low position
- Brachycephaly, in which the head is wider than it is longer

Medications & OSA

OSA may be brought on by or made worse by certain drugs. These include sedatives, narcotic-containing painkillers, and sleep aids. Drinking alcohol can have a comparable impact.

Hypothyroidism

Low thyroid hormone levels, or hypothyroidism, are a frequent medical issue that may raise the risk of OSA. It's critical to realize that treating hypothyroidism does not always cure OSA, which may require additional care.

Acromegaly

A uncommon medical condition called acromegaly is caused by pituitary tumors that oversecrete growth hormone. Adults with excessive growth hormone experience OSA due to the expansion of certain soft tissues and facial bones.

Muscle Diseases

Muscular dystrophy comes in a variety of forms. Some of these types put a person at higher risk of getting OSA.

Epidemiology of Obstructive Sleep Apnea

Since the fourth century BC, sleep apnea has been recognized throughout human history. Systematic research on individuals with obstructive sleep apnea hypopnea syndrome (OSAHS) and similar conditions replaced a number of publications from the 19th and early 20th centuries AD.34 Using methods created for the study of other disorders including narcolepsy and depression, OSAHS was first accurately established in neurophysiological sleep labs. Since OSAHS was first identified as such in 1965 35, facilities for diagnosis and treatment have grown dramatically, and knowledge of its far-reaching effects has advanced quickly.

Large-scale epidemiological studies have lately attempted to address difficulties with the incidence and prevalence of OSAHS, despite the fact that OSAHS was initially only described in case series. It is challenging to draw clear conclusions from these, though, because few of them have employed the finest techniques. The frequency of OSAHS in middle-aged males can be as high as 4%, according to the best-conducted research in terms of technique and process rigor 36. The study with the lowest reported prevalence may have inflated the incidence of OSAHS in the community by using oximetry alone because there were more than five 4% drops in arterial oxygen saturation detected by pulse oximetry per hour as a first screening test.37. However, by incorporating central apneas and breath-holds that occur during awake 38 using inductance plethysmography at home, those studies with the highest prevalences may have overstated the prevalence. Because each study used its own self-made questionnaires, the assessments of tiredness varied. There are fewer data on the prevalence of OSAHS in women, however it is likely half that of men (0.5–1%). 38

From newborns to the elderly, OSAHS affects people of all ages. The prevalence of respiratory disorders during sleep in adults rises with age and has little correlation with an increase in daytime tiredness or other OSAHS symptoms. 39

Because sleep apnea was considered a rare disorder in the early prevalence surveys, sleep recordings were only performed in sub-samples with a high probability of OSA in a first-stage screening method. The estimated prevalence in the general population was based on the presumption that the other participants had no OSA at all. In these investigations, the estimated prevalence of OSA syndrome varied between 0.7% and 3.3%.

Pathophysiology of Obstructive Sleep Apnea

The pathophysiological cause of OSA varies greatly from person to person. The anatomy of the upper airways, the ability of the upper airway dilator muscles to react to respiratory challenge during sleep, the tendency to awaken from increased respiratory drive during sleep (arousal threshold), the stability of the respiratory control system (loop gain), and the potential influence of state-related changes in lung volume are all probably significant factors.[40]

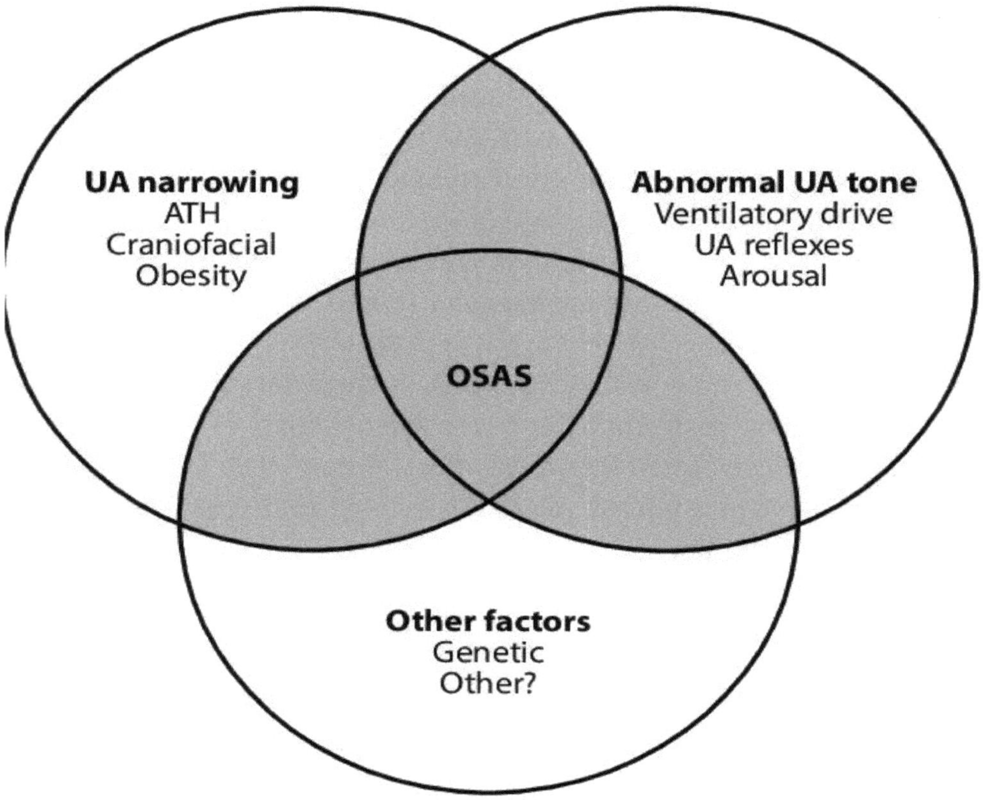

Fig 6: showing Pathophysiology of OSAS UPPER AIRWAY ANATOMY

The human upper airway is a special multipurpose structure that is used for breathing, speaking, and swallowing food and liquids. These diverse tasks are made possible by the evolution of the upper airway's architecture and neuronal regulation. As a result, the airway lacks hard or bony support and is made up of several muscles and soft tissues.

It has a foldable section that runs from the hard palate to the larynx, which is its most notable feature. Speech and swallowing during alertness depend on the upper airway's capacity to change form and briefly seal, but same ability also gives rise to collapse during inappropriate periods, like sleep.[41]

Anatomically speaking, a narrow upper airway is typically more likely to collapse than a broader one. Patients with OSA usually have a decreased cross-sectional area of the upper airway when they are awake compared to people without OSA, according to computed tomography and magnetic resonance imaging42. Additionally, OSA patients seem to have a distinct arrangement of surrounding soft tissues, which may increase the risk of upper airway collapse.[42]

Upper Airway Dilator Muscle Activity and Reflex Responsiveness

Patients with OSA seem to use defensive reflexes that increase upper airway dilator muscle activity to preserve airway patency during waking hours in order to compensate for a physically impaired upper airway.43. As a result, OSA patients have higher levels of activity in the genioglossus, the largest and most thoroughly researched upper airway dilator muscle in humans. One factor hypothesized to be important in the pathophysiology of OSA is the combination of pharyngeal anatomy and a reduced ability of the upper airway dilator muscles to maintain a patent airway during sleep 43. Multiunit EMG intramuscular electrodes of the genioglossus show that both healthy individuals and OSA patients have reduced muscle tone at the beginning of sleep, which lends credence to this notion.[44] Therefore, an individual who depends on muscle tone due to anatomic susceptibility will be especially vulnerable to developing OSA 45, even if healthy individuals suffer some degree of breathing instability and a drop of upper airway muscle tone at sleep start. As a result, hypopneas and apneas frequently happen when OSA patients go from awake to sleep. Thus, the improvement in apnea severity that is often observed in this sleep stage 46 when patients are able to reach slow wave sleep may be mostly due to greater activity of the upper airway dilator muscle. On the other hand, people with apnea might only be able to go into slow wave sleep when their breathing has stabilized and their muscle activity has risen.

Mechanistically, the genioglossus is significantly influenced by mechanoreceptive reflex processes that are locally mediated (i.e., in the upper airway) and react to negative pharyngeal pressure in addition to central respiratory drive.47. The genioglossus negative pressure reflex is one such mechanism that causes the muscle to contract in reaction to abrupt changes in negative intrapharyngeal pressure, or subatmospheric or suction pressure. 48. In healthy individuals, the genioglossus negative pressure reflex has been shown to decrease during non-REM sleep, which is consistent with the state-related nature of OSA.49. The identification of a supplementary state-dependent suppression component to this reflex arc suggests that decreased pharyngeal reflex responses during sleep may be mediated by more pronounced reflex inhibition rather than a loss of excitation. The genioglossus muscle clearly reacts to extended negative pressure and perhaps hypercapnia, particularly when many stimuli are given. The effectiveness of these compensatory reactions in restoring airflow during respiratory loading during sleep, however, appears to vary significantly.[50]

Arousal from Sleep

Arousal from sleep at the end of an apnea or hypopnea has long been thought to be an essential defense mechanism for reopening the airways. 51. Cortical arousal is linked to the majority of respiratory episodes, and more severe occurrences cause prolonged arousals.52. Younes has clarified the functional significance of arousal in OSA and disproved the notion that awakening from sleep is required for airway reopening.53. Younes demonstrated that when people with OSA were exposed to experimentally produced transient continuous positive airway pressure (CPAP) reductions, inspiratory flow increased in 22% of cases before to arousal and recovered in 17% of trials without arousal.[53] To investigate the mechanics behind these arousal-free recoveries of airflow, Jordan and associates undertook a study.50 Changes in duty cycle and an increase in genioglossus muscle activity were the outcomes of brief pressure drops lasting up to five minutes. Patients with OSA and healthy persons had similar compensatory reactions. However, compared to healthy individuals given stimuli of comparable amplitude, OSA patients were less able to restore breathing without cerebral arousal.

[50]Research indicates that patients with OSA can restore ventilation in the face of respiratory loading without cortical arousal at least occasionally, albeit to a lesser extent than healthy individuals. This suggests that some patients may be able to maintain a patent airway during sleep if they are able to stay asleep long enough to recruit compensatory mechanisms.

Ventilatory Control Stability

As previously mentioned, the development of a cyclical breathing pattern in which the patient cycles between arousal (wakefulness) and obstructive breathing events (sleep) is a typical feature of OSA. Furthermore, decreased respiratory drive is often associated with obstructive episodes. Therefore, it is thought that ventilatory control stability plays a significant role in the pathophysiology of OSA.

The engineering concept of loop gain can be used to characterize the stability of ventilatory regulation. 54. In essence, loop gain is the stability of a feedback loop-controlled system. Loop gain in ventilatory regulation refers to the respiratory system's stability and responsiveness to breathing disruptions, including arousal. Put differently, the tendency of the ventilatory control system to produce cyclical variations in ventilatory output (as observed in periodic breathing) is known as loop gain. Controller gain and plant gain are the two main parts of loop gain. Controller gain with relation to respiratory control describes the system's chemoresponsiveness(i.e., ventilatory responses to hypoxia and hypercapnia). The efficiency of $CO2$ excretion—that is, the capacity of a particular ventilation level to expel $CO2$—is the primary indicator of plant gain. Mixing gain, a third element that depends on both hemoglobin binding of $CO2$ and 02 and circulatory delay, seems to be less important. Mixing gain is frequently rather constant, though circulatory delays may make it more clinically relevant in people with congestive heart failure. 55 The ventilatory feedback control system is prone to instability due to the physical separation of the sensors and effectors. An innately high loop gain system (i.e., strong ventilatory response to a respiratory stimulus) is unstable in contrast to a low loop gain system.

(i.e., the reduced response of the ventilatory system to the same breathing input). The control of room temperature is a frequent example, where temperature oscillation may result from a too sensitive thermostat and an extremely powerful heater (i.e., high loop gain).

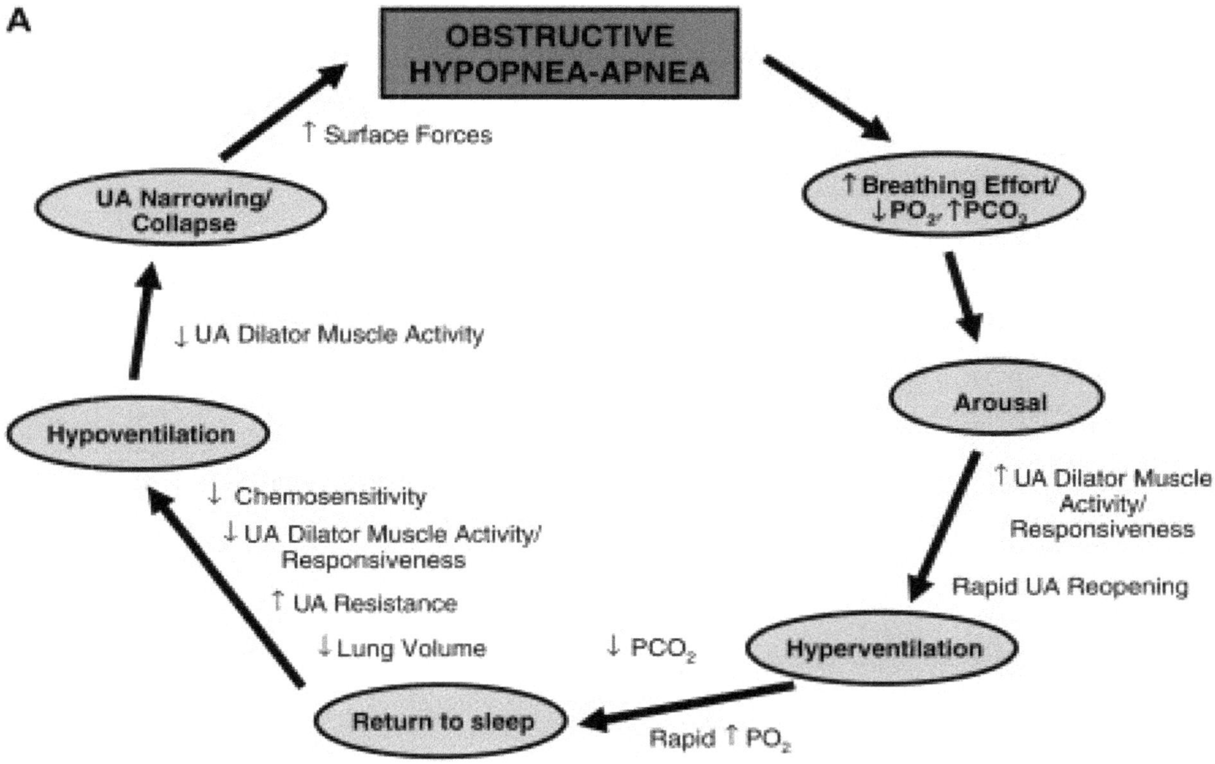

Proportional assist ventilation (PAV) is one method that has been developed to quantify loop gain of the respiratory system.

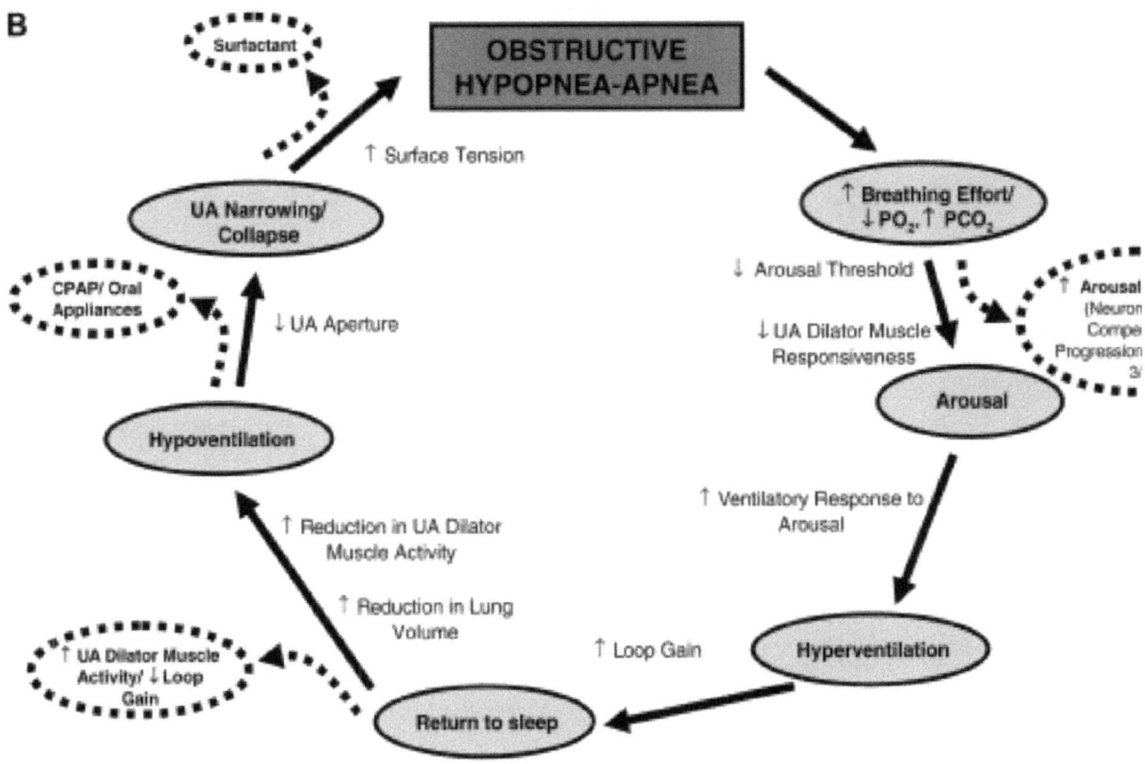

Figure 7 (shown in gray) graphically illustrates the typical pathophysiological sequence associated with obstructive sleep apnea (OSA), as well as the physiological processes that are either perpetuating (inside the circle) or protective/restorative (outside the circle) throughout the cycle. Upper airway is referred to as UA. (B) A schematic representation of the possible sites (within the main circle) where each of the several pathophysiological traits would either tend to exacerbate or predispose OSA. It should be mentioned that some of the effects of these traits may be related to one another (for instance, a large loop gain may cause periods of decreased upper airway dilator muscle activity as well as an increase in the ventilatory response to arousal and the predisposition for cyclical breathing). (A)

Friedman tongue Position

FTP is a straightforward method for estimating blockage at the hypopharyngeal level. Before FTP was developed, descriptions of hypopharyngeal blockage were inconsistent. Similar anatomical features were described using meaningless words like "retrognathia," "crowded oropharynx," and "macroglossia." Both patient care and data reporting are complicated by this.

The examination of the tongue's location with relation to the tonsils, pillars, hard palate, soft palate, and uvula is known as FTP. It is based on Mallampati phases, which are applied in anesthesiology when endotracheal intubation is challenging. The Mallampati system has three grades and examines the palate with the tongue protruded, while FTP evaluates the palate with the tongue in a neutral position inside the mouth. Additionally, FTP II is divided into IIa and IIb, and FTP is assigned on a scale from I to IV.[56]

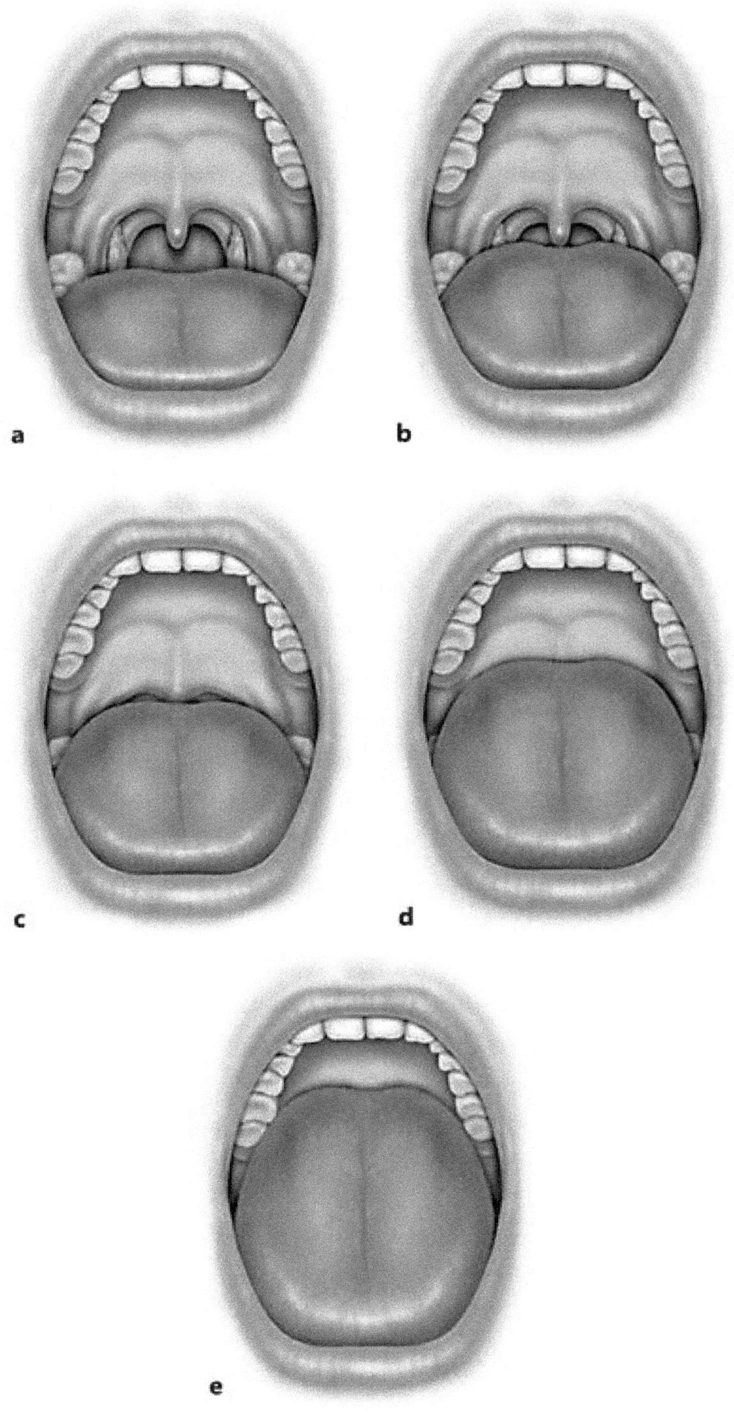

Fig 8 Showing Friedman tongue position (FTP). a FTP I visualizes the uvula and tonsils/pillar.

b The tonsils and pillar are not visible in FTP IIa, but the majority of the uvula is. The entire soft palate up to the uvular base can be seen with FTP IIb. A portion of the soft palate is seen in FTP III, but the distal end is missing. Only the hard palate is seen in FTP IV.

Obesity and Obstructive Sleep Apnea

One significant risk factor for OSA is obesity. Up to 70% of those who are severely obese have OSA.[57]

Due to fat buildup in specific areas, obesity may make OSA worse. Fat accumulation in the tissues surrounding the upper airway seems to predispose people to apnea by narrowing the lumen and making the upper airway more collapsible.58. Furthermore, truncal obesity, or fat accumulation around the thorax, lowers functional residual capacity and chest compliance and may raise oxygen demand.59. Individuals with OSA frequently have visceral obesity. Sixty Furthermore, truncal obesity, or fat accumulation around the thorax, lowers functional residual capacity and chest compliance and may raise oxygen demand. [57] Individuals with OSA frequently have visceral obesity.58. But the connection between obesity and OSA is nuanced. Recent research indicates that OSA may itself lead to weight increase, despite strong evidence that obesity, including visceral obesity, may contribute to OSA and that decreasing weight improves OSA. 61. Weight gain in OSA patients may be caused by factors including decreased activity levels and increased appetite, especially for refined carbs. 62. It is still unknown whether OSA predisposes to preferred visceral fat accumulation. 63 CPAP treatment for OSA lowers visceral fat (as evaluated by abdominal CT scanning). even in individuals who haven't lost a lot of weight. 64 Patel et al. found a substantial association (range from 0.57 to 0.61) between anthropomorphic adiposity measurements and AHI, indicating that obesity may account for roughly 40% of the genetic diversity in sleep apnea.65. In a different study, Popko et al. demonstrated a strong correlation between OSA and obesity when compared to healthy controls and polymorphisms of the leptin receptor, which is involved in energy balance and body weight regulation (Arg/Arg and Gln/Arg when compared with Gln/Gln).[66]

These findings imply that genetic polymorphisms may have an impact on obesity and sleep apnea and may play a significant role in their development.

Diagnosis of Obstructive Sleep Apnea

Nocturnal polysomnography (PSG) is the gold standard for diagnosing pediatric OSA when the history and exam are suspicious. However, using a PSG for evaluation can be costly, time-consuming, and resource-constrained. A PSG is still necessary for the diagnosis of OSA, although overnight oximetry at home can be utilized as a technique to provide additional information. 67. If an underlying cardiovascular problem is suspected, a chest x-ray and EKG are also required for additional evaluation. If required, an echocardiogram may be included in the cardiac workup; this is especially important for kids with severe OSA prior to surgery. It may also be more beneficial to measure a number of inflammatory biomarkers that can be elevated in children with OSA, such as kallikrein-1, uromodulin, urocortin-3, and orosomucoid-1. It is also appropriate to perform TSH, iron tests, and a complete blood count (CBC) in order to look into other significant causes of sleep disturbance. Imaging methods are only helpful in conjunction with a PSG to offer a conclusive diagnosis, although they can evaluate underlying anatomic abnormalities that may contribute to OSA.[69]

Certain aspects of sleep amount and quality are monitored during PSG. Blood oxygen levels, eye and limb movements, brain activity, heart rate, nasal and oral air movement, and snoring are all measured by sensors. Calculations like sleep efficiency, sleep onset latency, and time spent in each stage of sleep are made possible by the data gathered. A PSG measures the apnea/hypopnea index (AHI), which is the average of the apneic and hypopneic events per hour of sleep and is essential for the diagnosis of OSA. If the AHI score is between 1 and 4.9 events per hour, OSA is considered mild; if it is between 5 and 9.9 events per hour, it is considered moderate; and if it is greater than 9 events per hour, it is considered severe.66 There is some debate on the clinical importance of an AHI of 1 to 1.9 events/hour, however an AHI of 1 or more is abnormal in children up to the age of 13. Seventy. Depending on the patient's development and clinical picture, either pediatric or adult criteria may be applied between the ages of 13 and 17. Children's PSG is typically characterized by hypopneic episodes rather than outright apnea because of their better airway integrity and lower likelihood of collapse compared to adults.

It's interesting to note that hypercarbia, which is absent in the adult OSA population, may also be present in the pediatric population when diagnosing pediatric OSA. This is less prevalent in adults and is brought on by a protracted hypoventilation state.[66]

Diagnostic criteria

The updated International Classification of Sleep Disorders, Third Edition (ICSD-3) 71 (A and B) or C satisfies the following criteria:

A. **The presence of one or more of the following**

- The patient reports feeling exhausted, having trouble falling asleep, having insomnia, or having restless nights.
- The patient wakes up clutching their breath, gasping, or choking.
- Regular snoring or breathing disruptions during sleep are reported by the bed mate or an observer.
- The patient has type 2 diabetes mellitus, congestive heart failure, atrial fibrillation, coronary artery disease, stroke, hypertension, a mental problem, or cognitive impairment.

B. **Polysomnography (PSG) or out-of-center sleep testing (OCST) demonstrates**

Five or more predominantly obstructive respiratory events (obstructive apneas, hypopneas, or respiratory effort related arousals [RERAs]) must occur per hour of sleep during a PSG or an OCST.

C. **PSG or OCST demonstrates**

During a PSG or monitoring (OCST), 15 or more primarily obstructive respiratory episodes (hypopneas, apneas, or RERAs) occur every hour of sleep.

Definition or Scoring of Respiratory Events During PSG

The criteria outlined in the AASM Manual for the Scoring of Sleep and Associated episodes are used to describe and score different respiratory episodes in adults.[72]

If the respiratory effort signal drops by at least 90% of the pre-event baseline for at least 10 seconds and the inspiratory effort from the chest and/or abdomen continues or increases, it is considered obstructive apnea.A hypopnea is characterized by a decrease in respiratory effort of at least 30% of the pre-event baseline for at least 10 seconds, accompanied by oxygen desaturation of at least 3% (AASM criteria) or 4% (CMS criteria).

If the inspiratory nasal pressure flattens for more than ten seconds, resulting in an arousal from sleep but not matching the criteria for apnea or hypopnea, the condition is called Respiratory Effort-Related Arousal (RERA).

- The indices used to measure the severity of OSA include the Apnea Hypopnea Index (AHI), the Respiratory Disturbance Index (RDI) if PSG is performed, or the Respiratory Event Index (REI) if OCST is performed. The AHI is calculated by dividing the total sleep time by the number of apneas and hypopneas.
- The number of apneas, hypopneas, and RERAs divided by the total amount of sleep time yields the RDI.
- REI is calculated by dividing the total number of apneas and hypopneas by the duration of monitoring.

- For adults, AHI or REI <5/hour is considered normal; 5–14.9/hour is considered mild OSA; 15–29.9/hour is considered moderate OSA; and ≥30/hour is considered severe OSA.Signs and Symptoms of OSA

The most prevalent symptoms in OSA patients are snoring and daytime tiredness. Other symptoms during the night include nocturia, erectile dysfunction, frequent arousals, restless sleep, waking up choking or gasping, and apneas that the bedpartner witnesses. OSA patients may have unrefreshing sleep, headaches in the morning, low energy, difficulty concentrating, exhaustion, or a negative mood.

OSA has been linked to inattention, decreased productivity, and traffic or workplace accidents. OSA doubles or triples the likelihood of a car accident. Treatment for OSA, such as continuous positive airway pressure (CPAP) therapy, can significantly lower this risk.[73]

According to American Academy of Pediatric Dentistry (2012) Signs and symptoms of OSAS: -

Excessive daytime sleepiness
Loud snoring three or more nights per week
Episodes of breathing cessation witnessed by another person.
Abrupt awakenings accompanied by shortness of breath.

Awakening with dry mouth or sore throat.
Morning headache
Difficulty staying asleep
Attention problems
Mouth breathing
Sweating
Restlessness
Waking up a lot

Examination of patient

The Body Mass Index (BMI) should be measured because obesity is a significant risk factor for OSA. An increased risk of OSA is linked to a neck circumference of at least 17 inches in men and 16 inches in women. Macroglossia, enlarged tonsils, large uvula, retrognathia, nasal septal deviation, and turbinate hypertrophy are examples of upper airway anomalies that increase the risk of OSA. The Mallampati score can be used to clinically quantify airway constriction. [74].

The following is the updated Mallampati score that is currently widely used:

- Class 0: Any visible portion of the epiglottis
- Class I: visible pillars, uvula, and soft palate
- Class II: visible uvula and soft palate
- Class III: Only the base of the uvula and the soft palate are visible
- Class IV: Only the hard palate is visible

A patient must be seated upright, open their mouth, and extend their tongue as much as possible in order for their Mallampati score to be appropriately determined. This exam is often administered without phonation.[74]

Clinical significance of Mallampati score:

In order to forecast the difficult airway, the Mallampati score system was introduced in the 1980s and soon became a standard preoperative physical examination. Based on the laryngeal views reported in the initial study, early research found that Class III and IV could predict difficult intubation. 74. However, Mallampati's initial study's laryngeal views did not align with the most widely used Cormack-Lehane grading system, which was described a year after his suggested indication.

Screening Tools for obstructive sleep apnea

Several screening methods, including the Berlin questionnaire, STOP-BANG questionnaire, and preoperative questionnaire, are used to identify people who are at risk. One popular instrument for OSA screening is the Epworth Tiredness Scale (ESS), a subjective indicator of weariness. STOPBANG is a very sensitive, user-friendly gadget. While patients with scores between 5 and 8 have a considerable likelihood of developing moderate to severe OSA (AHI >15), individuals with scores between 0 and 2 have a minimal chance of developing OSA.[75]

STOP BANG score

	Question	**Yes or No**
S	Do you **Snore** loudly?	
T	Do you feel **Tired** or sleepy during the day?	
O	Has anyone **Observed** apneas or choking during sleep?	
P	Do you have high Blood **Pressure**	
B	**BMI** > 35	
A	**Age** > 50	
N	**Neck** circumference ≥17 inches (men); ≥16 inches (women)	
G	**Gender** – male	

Table 5: Stop Bang Score [75]

Diagnostic Tests

The number of channels that are examined during the test determines how sleep tests are categorized. The gold standard for diagnosing OSA is the type 1 test, often known as polysomnography (PSG) or an in-lab attended sleep study. At-home sleep testing or out-of-center sleep testing (OCST)

When PSG is not practical, the Apnea Test (HSAT), a type 3 test, is a good substitute. Since there is no EEG recording, the HSAT cannot measure sleep. Following a thorough sleep assessment, AASM recommends HSAT for people with high pretest chance. HSAT should not be used as a screening tool in patients who also have severe pulmonary disease, congestive heart failure, neuromuscular disease, or other sleep disorders such parasomnias, narcolepsy, or periodic limb movement disorder (PLMD). When a patient with symptoms and a high index of suspicion for OSA has a negative or technically insufficient HSAT, an in-lab PSG should be performed.

Clinical Manifestations of Obstructive Sleep Apnea

The symptoms of obstructive sleep apnea (OSA) can range from mild interference with day-to-day activities to extreme drowsiness, snoring, observed apneas, and other typical symptoms. OSA is still underdiagnosed despite mounting evidence that it can negatively impact health in a number of ways. The cardiovascular system is one among OSA's most well-documented health effects. The severity of the symptoms frequently worsens over years, delaying identification and giving the illness more time to negatively impact health.

In order to correctly identify patients at risk for the disease, conduct the necessary tests, and customize therapy for each patient, clinicians should be knowledgeable about both the subtle and overt clinical signs of OSA.

OSA is strongly associated with hypertension and arrhythmias, and research indicates that treating OSA may be especially crucial for individuals with resistant hypertension and those undergoing cardioversion for atrial fibrillation. There have also been well-documented significant correlations between heart failure and both complicated sleep apnea and OSA. OSA is also linked to poorly regulated mood disorder, cerebrovascular injury, and decreased neurocognition. Treatment for OSA may slow the advancement of atherosclerosis and enhance outcomes following a cerebrovascular accident (CVA).

Patients with extreme sleepiness as a component of their co-morbid mood problems, actual or near-miss auto accidents, and complaints of poor focus at work should all be evaluated for OSA.

There has also been research on the metabolic effects of OSA, especially with regard to glucose homeostasis. Because untreated OSA negatively affects lipid levels and glucose tolerance, it has been suggested that OSA is another component of the metabolic syndrome. The detrimental consequences of untreated OSA on liver health may be connected to some of these metabolic abnormalities.

Cardiovascular association

Perhaps the most well-established consequence of OSA is lower cardiovascular outcomes. Although many cardiovascular risk factors (male sex, age, obesity, hypertension, and glucose intolerance) are prevalent in the OSA community, elevated risk is independently associated with OSA. It is commonly known that sleep apnea and cardiovascular disease have a dangerous connection.

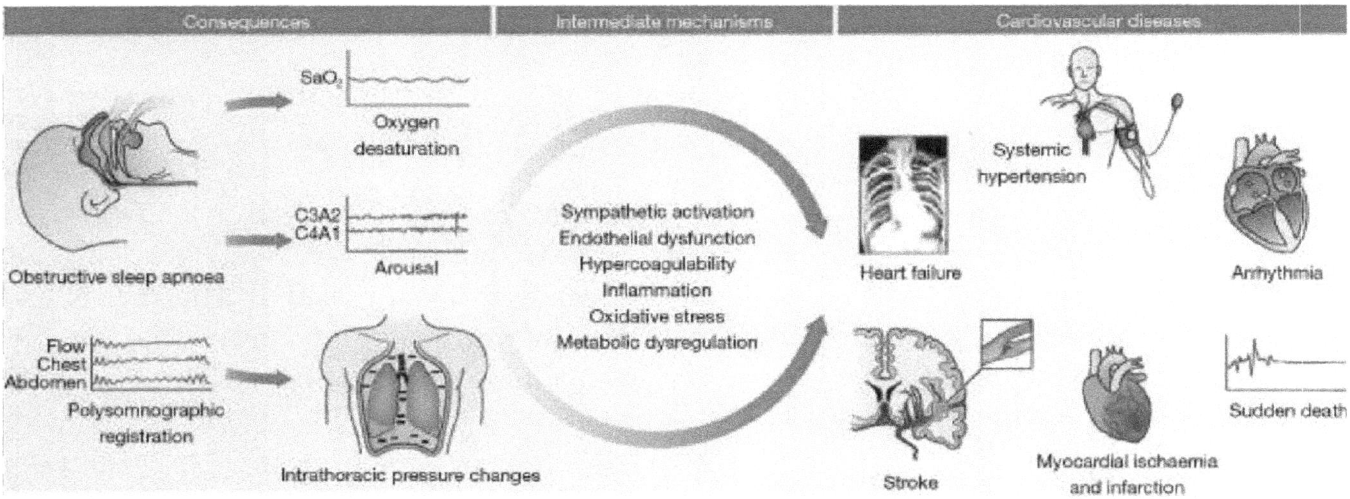

Fig 9 showing Pathological relationship between sleep apnea and cardiovascular disease [76] OSA and hypertension

It was first proposed more than 30 years ago that OSA and hypertension were related.77 There is substantial debate regarding the present body of research that links OSA to the onset of hypertension. Patients at a particular severity of OSA are probably susceptible to developing hypertension in different ways. The research that is now available indicates that CPAP therapy can improve blood pressure, albeit only slightly. Nevertheless, it is unlikely that CPAP therapy will have a clinically meaningful effect on a patient with mild sleep apnea who is asymptomatic.

OSA and Arrythmias

The OSA population has a long history of arrhythmias, especially atrial fibrillation, which are probably caused by respiratory irregularities and altered autonomic tone during sleep. The association between OSA and cardiac arrhythmia is supported by both recent case-control and cross-sectional research and studies that go back more than 30 years.78.

Among the rhythm problems discovered during these tests are ventricular tachycardia or fibrillation, sinus arrest, atrioventricular conduction blocks, complex ventricular ectopy, supraventricular tachycardia, bradycardia, and atrial fibrillation.[77]

Sleep Disorders breathing (SDB) and OSA

Pure OSA or central apnea with Cheynne-Stokes respiration are two common manifestations of SDB in the heart failure population. When Javaheri assessed 81 ambulatory males with congestive heart failure in 1998, he reported this connection. 79 There appears to be a reciprocal association between SDB and CHF, with one aggravating the other.

Pulmonary hypertension and OSA

Another cardiovascular condition that has a clear connection to OSA is pulmonary hypertension (PH). OSA was added to group 3 of the World Health Organization's PH categorization system (PH related to lung illnesses and/or hypoxia) as a result of this relationship. Eighty One would anticipate that treatment for OSA patients with positive airway pressure would only slightly lower PAP given the slight rise in pulmonary arterial pressure caused by OSA. [80].

Another cardiovascular condition that is strongly associated with OSA is pulmonary hypertension (PH). OSA was placed in group 3 of the World Health Organization's PH categorization system (PH connected to lung diseases and/or hypoxia) as a result of this association. Eighty One would anticipate that treatment for OSA patients with positive airway pressure would only slightly reduce PAP given the slight increase in pulmonary artery pressure caused by OSA.[78].

Neurocognitive associations

Stroke is the most well-documented neurologic consequence that also coincides with the cardiovascular effects of OSA. Stroke can result from the aforementioned cardiovascular effects of OSA, such as atrial fibrillation, heart failure, and hypertension. Patients who have had a stroke may experience better clinical results if they receive treatment for SDB. Different levels of neurocognitive impairment are linked to OSA.

These neurocognitive impairments in the OSA population can be surrogately detected in a clinic through work performance deficiencies and traffic accidents. OSA is frequently linked to cerebrovascular injury and poor neurocognition. Treatment for OSA may lessen the progression of atherosclerosis and improve outcomes after a CVA. Patients should be evaluated for OSA if they have experienced actual or near-miss traffic accidents, report difficulty concentrating at work, or exhibit extreme fatigue as part of their co-morbid mood condition.

Metabolic associations

The research that is now available indicates that OSA adversely impacts people's metabolic profiles, particularly in cases of moderate-to-severe disease. OSA may be a component of metabolic syndrome due to its negative impact on glucose homeostasis, fatty liver disease, and lipid metabolism.81. OSA affects the metabolism of glucose. Changes in the hypothalamic-pituitary-adrenal axis, aberrant sympathetic activation, the synthesis of certain adipokines, and increased inflammation/oxidative stress caused by SDB have been identified as the intermediary mechanisms between OSA and altered glucose metabolism. Eighty The connection between OSA and diabetes is still up for debate because OSA's physiological abnormalities are known to change glucose metabolism. Glycemic control appears to be somewhat improved by correcting apneic episodes with positive airway pressure.

Liver steatosis is a recognized indicator of insulin resistance and metabolic syndrome. Recent research has examined how OSA affects individuals with the metabolic syndrome and the development of nonalcoholic fatty liver disease (NAFLD), nonalcoholic steatohepatitis (NASH), asymptomatic hepatic steatosis, and eventually cirrhotic liver disease.

OSA and Craniofacial and Dentofacial Development

OSA is linked to specific craniofacial characteristics. An inferiorly and posteriorly positioned hyoid on cephalometry and an elevated anterior face height have been linked to a higher risk of OSA.

Although there was more variation and heterogeneity between studies, OSA was similarly linked to acute anterior cranial base angles, lower anterior cranial base length, shorter maxillary and mandibular length, and higher posterior rotation of the jaw. Transverse face dimensions of people with and without OSA have been compared using three-dimensional imaging, revealing that those with OSA have more arched palates and smaller interdental widths.

Management of Pediatric Obstructive Sleep Apnea

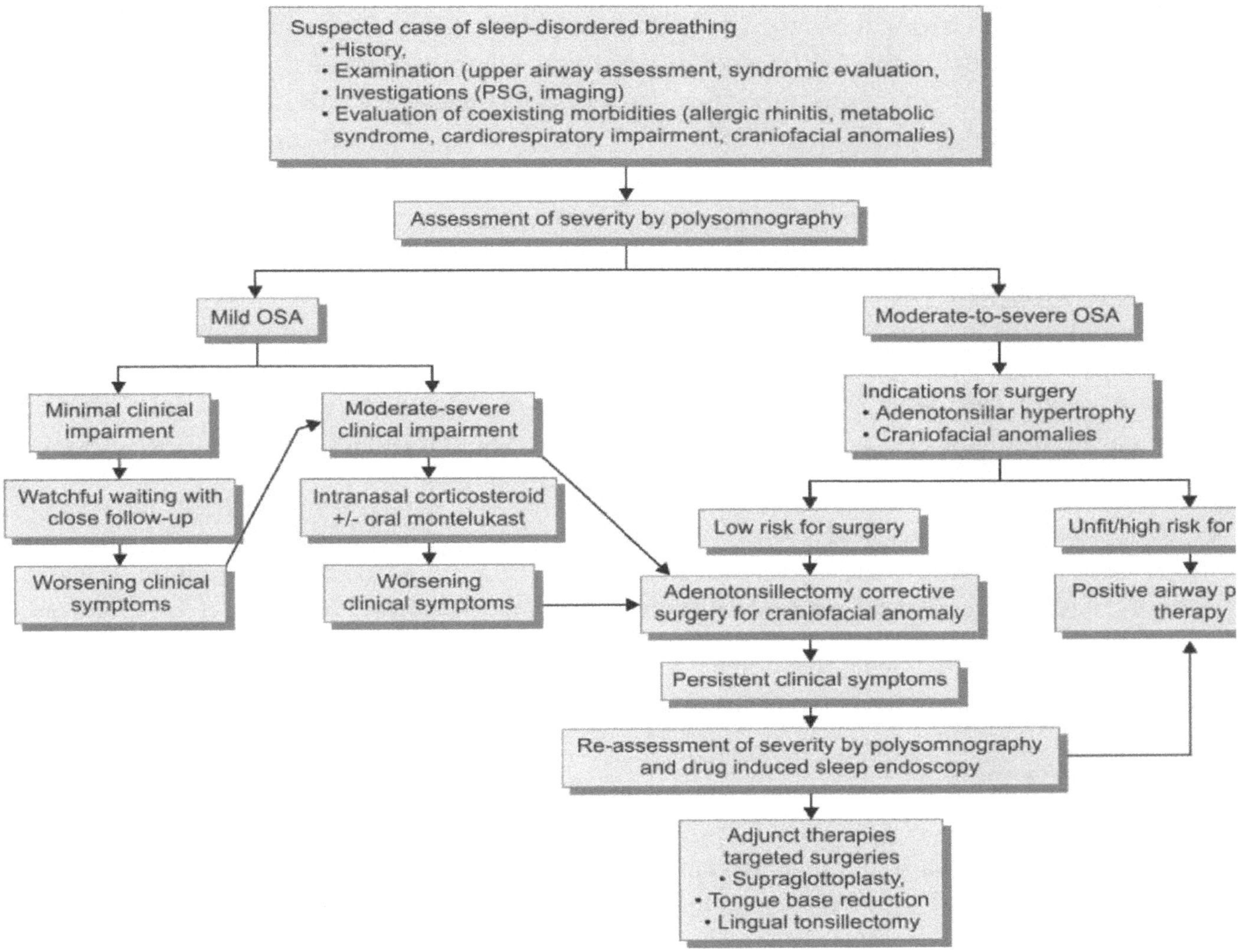

Fig 10: Over the past 20 years, treatment strategies for children obstructive sleep apnea (OSA) have significantly changed. Depending on how severe the OSA is, there are numerous treatment options. These consist of both non-surgical and surgical procedures.

Non-Surgical management of obstructive sleep apnea

Pediatric patients with mild to severe OSA may benefit from a leukotriene inhibitor (montelukast) treatment study. 82 After three months of treatment, montelukast has been demonstrated to drastically reduce adenotonsillar size, which in suitable patients results in a reduction in AHI. 81 Pediatric OSA cannot be effectively treated with systemic glucocorticoids. On the other hand, patients with mild to severe OSA may benefit from intranasal steroid treatment for six weeks, which has been demonstrated to improve the AHI.[67]

Most patients will experience a clinically meaningful reduction in AHI when intranasal steroids and leukotriene inhibitors are used. 83 Up to six months of "watchful waiting" may be suitable for patients with mild to moderate OSA. This is typically done in an effort to address underlying issues that could improve OSA and AHI without the need for surgery, such as obesity or allergic rhinitis. However, A&T is better at improving the AHI in pediatric patients who are not obese or syndromic. Another possible course of treatment is continuous positive airway pressure, or CPAP. Although PAP is the first-line treatment for adults, its usage in children has certain restrictions. If the child is not a suitable candidate for surgery or if they still have moderate to severe OSA after surgery, PAP should be taken into consideration during the perioperative phase before A&T for severe OSA. Participation may be challenging for kids, and wearing the same mask over and over again may change the anatomy of the face. Oral appliances (OAs) have been shown to lower AHI in adults, but there aren't enough studies on pediatric populations to assess their efficacy or identify which kids might benefit from them.82.A novel approach to treating OSA in both adults and children is myofunctional therapy. In addition to proper tongue positioning, this requires retraining the oropharyngeal structures and oral cavity muscles. Research on children with OSA is scarce, and little is known about its effectiveness. However, this could be a subject for additional research and used as an OSA supplement.[84]

Patients who have a reversible risk factor for OSA, particularly obesity, should receive counseling on how to reverse the condition. Losing weight can help with OSA can be used as an additional treatment for older kids. 82 Parents should be counseled to restrict their children's exposure to tobacco use and secondhand smoke at home.

Non-surgical management of obstructive sleep apne

High flow nasal cannula

Treatment of obstructive sleep apnea without surgery Nasal cannula with high flow In certain research, high flow nasal cannulas have demonstrated potential as a CPAP substitute 85. This treatment involves continuously supplying the upper airway with humidified air through a soft plastic nasal cannula.

A few modest studies have shown statistically significant improvements in AHI with high flow nasal cannulas thus far. Airway stenting, heat and humidity-induced congestion reduction, and stimulation of upper airway tone 85 are some theories regarding its effectiveness, while the exact mechanism is unknown. Younger OSA patients and those who are intolerant to CPAP may benefit from this treatment, even if more thorough research is needed to evaluate the mechanism and effectiveness of high flow nasal cannulas.

Oxygen therapy

Airflow restriction and subsequent oxygen desaturation result from partial or total obstruction of the upper airway in OSA.

Because it is thought to alter the respiratory response (loop gain) to hypoxemia86, supplemental oxygen has been utilized to treat desaturations. Oxygen treatment has become particularly popular for infants because CPAP is not FDA-approved for anyone under 13 kg. In a retrospective investigation of 23 neonates, the infusion of 0.25–1.0 L/min of additional oxygen during the second half of a split-night sleep study significantly increased total oxygen saturation, oxygen nadir, and AHI.

Positional therapy

It has been demonstrated that OSA is worse in supine individuals. The tongue slipping into the oropharynx is most likely the mechanism that makes obstructive episodes worse. Medical-made back cushions and padding, as well as improvised items like tennis balls sewed to the back of a shirt or a backpack worn while sleeping, are devices designed to keep people sleeping in a lateral position with the ultimate goal of making supine sleep difficult. There are now neck-worn devices that vibrate when a patient rolls off their side in an attempt to change their behavior.[87]

Watchful waiting

Factors that contribute to OSA, including as obesity, neuromuscular tone, and allergies, might gradually improve during the pediatric population's period of continuous growth and development. Patients were randomly assigned to either early adenotonsillectomy [28] or vigilant waiting in the CHAT (Childhood Adenotonsillectomy Trial). Interestingly, 46% of kids in the watchful waiting group also saw their AHI return to normal without any surgery, while 79% of children who underwent adenotonsillectomy experienced remission of their OSA. Obesity, African American race, and an AHI higher than the study's median of 4.7 events/h were factors linked to OSA non-resolution following watchful waiting. Therefore, when counseling patients with mild OSA who do not have severe comorbidities, watchful waiting is a significant alternative.

Surgical management of obstructive sleep apnea Adenotonsillectomy (T&A)

Undoubtedly, hypertrophy of upper airway lymphadenoid tissues is the most common cause of children's obstructive sleep apnea (OSA), which was only formally identified as a separate condition in 1976 by Guilleminault and collaborators.3The American Academy of Pediatrics (AAP) consensus guidelines for pediatric OSA in 2002 and 2012 recommended adenotonsillectomy (T&A) as the initial treatment due to this commonly confirmed finding. 87. In actuality, up to 75% of higher-risk groups, such as obese children, may experience residual OSA after T&A, although 13% to 29% of children categorized as low-risk patients may experience persistent OSA. 88 Other risk factors for OSA persistence after surgery include age greater than seven years, asthma, nocturnal enuresis, allergic rhinitis, and the severity of OSA prior to T&A.85 Increased collapsibility of the upper airways is often brought on by changes in neural reflexes, inappropriate recruitment of the upper airway musculature, or local inflammation, such as asthma or allergic rhinitis. individuals suffering from neuromuscular diseases or cerebral palsy. Most OSA patients usually have more than one contributing factor. The majority of patients are unlikely to be treated by T&A alone due to the usually complex pathophysiology of juvenile OSA.

Lingual tonsillectomy

The tongue has a major role in the pathophysiology of OSA. Macroglossia and glossoptosis result in a posteriorly positioned tongue that is more likely to collapse into the airway during sleep.89.

This is observed in OSA-causing disorders such Beckwith-Wiedemann syndrome, Pierre-Robin sequence, and Down syndrome. Similar to the growth of the palatine tonsils or adenoids, lingual tonsil hypertrophy can also happen. To lessen the severity of posterior tongue collapse, tongue base reduction surgery entails surgically removing the lingual tonsils along with or without a piece of the posterior tongue musculature.[89].

Supraglottoplasty

Excessively redundant or floppy upper airway tissue that causes blockage is a congenital disease known as laryngomalacia90. It is a known cause of OSA in this age group and usually manifests as stridor in newborns and babies. Congenital laryngomalacia usually gets better as the patient gets older, and surgery is only performed on patients who show severe respiratory distress or failure to thrive. A surgical procedure called supraglottoplasty removes extra upper airway tissue to prevent collapse. [90].

Tracheostomy

A tracheostomy is the surgical insertion of a tube from the midline neck through an incision into the trachea. One effective treatment for OSA91 that completely prevents upper airway collapse is tracheostomy. Children with craniofacial anomalies or neuromuscular dysfunction who are not responding to alternative treatment modalities are often the most severe and resistant patients for whom tracheostomy has been used. Despite its therapeutic benefits, tracheostomy is linked to long-term problems include recurrent infections, unintentional decannulation, and even death. There is also a corresponding decline in living quality. Additionally, tracheostomy care places a greater care burden on the family92. Because of these factors, tracheostomy is still a very uncommon therapeutic option for pediatric OSA. When deciding whether to pursue this therapy, healthcare professionals should consider the severity of the disease burden as well as the risks associated with the procedure.

Newer diagnostic and treatment modalities in pediatric OSA

The key to identifying juvenile OSA is PSG, a multichannel sleep recording that typically occurs in a licensed sleep laboratory. OSA severity is classified as mild, moderate, or severe using the obstructive apnea-hypopnea index (AHI).87. Even while flow restrictions, respiratory effort, and oxygen desaturation during polysomnography are used to diagnose OSA, these parameters only partially reflect the upper airway collapse. Regular polysomnography does not visualize the upper airway during collapse. Two techniques used to help observe and determine the degree and type of upper airway collapse in patients with OSA are drug-induced sleep endoscopy (DISE) and cine magnetic resonance imaging (Cine MRI).[87].

During the **DISE** procedure, a flexible endoscope is inserted via the nose to view the upper airway while sedatives are administered to the patient. The upper airway will collapse as the patient becomes more sedated but breathes on their own; this is believed to be related to the collapse that takes place during sleep. This method is being used more frequently, particularly in kids who still have OSA following an adenotonsillectomy.[93].

Cine MRI uses a series of MRI pictures to show the upper airway in real time. It is better than DISE because it makes the entire upper airway visible.

Nevertheless, there is little research on whether Cine MRI has improved surgical outcomes or helped direct treatments. Patients must lie still in a machine for an extended amount of time in order to obtain MRI images, which is a challenging and time-consuming procedure. For this operation, children must be sedated, which raises the question of whether sedation actually replicates sleep. [94].

Treatment of Residual OSA

For children with moderate to severe OSA following T&A, non-invasive positive airway pressure (PAP) therapy has unquestionably been the most often chosen course of treatment, along with anti-inflammatory medication. Nevertheless, a number of emerging therapies have started to be investigated and should also be discussed.

- **Weight Loss:**

  As a possible treatment for OSA and because weight loss improves both short-term and long-term morbidity in juvenile obesity, efforts to encourage weight loss in obese children with residual OSA should be encouraged. Dietary therapies aimed at promoting weight loss or at least minimum weight gain were used to treat obese children with mild OSA who did not exhibit physical signs of adenotonsillar hypertrophy in the NANOS experiment, a multicenter trial on obesity and OSA conducted in Spain.[95]

- **Positive Airway Pressure Therapy:**

  PAP therapy is commonly utilized as a primary intervention for children who do not have enlarged tonsils and adenoids or to treat children who exhibit moderate to severe OSA following T&A. The main benefits of PAP include maintaining airway patency during the respiratory cycle while you're asleep, improving functional residual capacity (FRC), and lowering the effort required to breathe due to elevated airway resistance 96. CPAP is used in the great majority of patientsBilevel PAP therapy may be required for patients who require extremely high positive end expiratory pressures or who have medical conditions such as obesity hypoventilation syndrome or neuromuscular diseases in order to achieve the ultimate goal of normalizing gas exchange abnormalities and enabling restorative and continuous sleep throughout the night. Despite the obvious advantages of PAP therapy, there are a few issues and worries that should be mentioned in addition to poor adherence. Abdominal distension, oronasal dryness, eye irritation, nasal bridge pressure sores from the masks, and general pain from air leaks are common. Additionally, when PAP is applied at a very young age, the mask's prolonged pressure on developing facial features may cause flattening of the midface or maxillary retrusion, which must be closely observed via digital photography. [96].

- **Drug Induced Sleep Endoscopy:**

  Imaging techniques have evolved and are being utilized increasingly often in clinical settings in an attempt to better forecast the overall effects of T&A or to specify an appropriate therapy approach for children with residual OSA. Drug-induced sleep endoscopy (DISE) allows upper airway exploration by inserting a flexible fiberoptic endoscope through the nose during spontaneous breathing while the patient is under conscious sedation. DISE's primary goals are to replicate upper airway circumstances as nearly as possible to those that arise during normal sleep.[97]

- **Rapid Maxillary Expansion**

  The idea that more intraoral and upper airway introitus space will reduce airflow resistance and improve airway patency has led to the development of methods for facilitating rapid maxillary expansion (RME) over many years. RME usually consists of a fixed appliance with an expansion system attached to opposing teeth that is gradually used to extend the midpalatal suture in order to enhance the transverse diameter of the hard palate over a period of weeks to months. Reducing or eliminating children's residual OSA is one of the intervention's clear theoretical benefits.[98].

- **Isolated Obstructive Hypoventilation**

  The term "obstructive alveolar hypoventilation," which describes a prevalent issue in children who snore, was initially used by Rosen and associates. 98. It has been demonstrated that certain kids who are categorized as primary snorers also occasionally and consistently have elevated CO2 levels. However, the relationship between overnight end-tidal carbon dioxide levels and other polysomnographic data is quite weak. Additionally, obstructive hypoventilation usually improves with T&A; however, the degree of hypoventilation improvement is not associated with behavioral or cognitive changes after surgery, and these improvements are not as predictive of the clinical response as AHI.[99]

Oral appliances given to children with OSA

Functional orthopaedic appliances are often removable intraoral devices that modify the stresses exerted by the muscles against the teeth and the maxilla and mandible, which make up the facial skeleton.

These are dynamic appliances that influence occlusal development and bone formation by modified neuromuscular action 100.

Oral appliances for sleep apnea are mouthpieces or dental gadgets that patients wear in their mouths to maintain an open airway while they sleep. They are used by medical professionals to treat obstructive sleep apnea (OSA).

When a patient has OSA, their upper airway may be partially or totally obstructed while they sleep. The brain awakens the patient just enough to continue breathing as a result of the decreased airflow. Throughout the night, the cycle of restricted airflow, waking, and falling back asleep persists.

These episodes prohibit the patient from obtaining enough oxygen to their important organs and prevent them from sleeping soundly. OSA is potentially lethal and can cause major health issues if left untreated.

OSA is treated with oral appliances, often known as oral appliance therapy. They hold the patient's mouth in a way that ensures adequate ventilation. They improve the patient's breathing and lessen the frequency of OSA awakenings.

Types of oral appliances used to treat obstructive sleep apnea (OSA)

Mandibular advancement devices (MADs) and tongue-stabilizing devices (TSDs) are the two primary categories of dental appliances used to treat OSA.

Mandibular advancement devices

The most popular dental appliance for treating OSA is a mandibular advancement device (MAD). They are also known as mandibular repositioning appliances, mandibular advancement appliances, or mandibular advancement splints.

Your lower jaw, or mandible, is pulled forward by MADs. Your tongue is drawn forward when you move your jaw forward, which increases the amount of airflow in the back of your throat. MADs cover your teeth. The majority are divided into two sections: one for your upper teeth and one for your lower teeth. You can move the lower portion of the gadget that controls your jaw forward by using screws, hinges, and modified rubber bands to link the top and bottom. Others have separate, interchangeable arches.

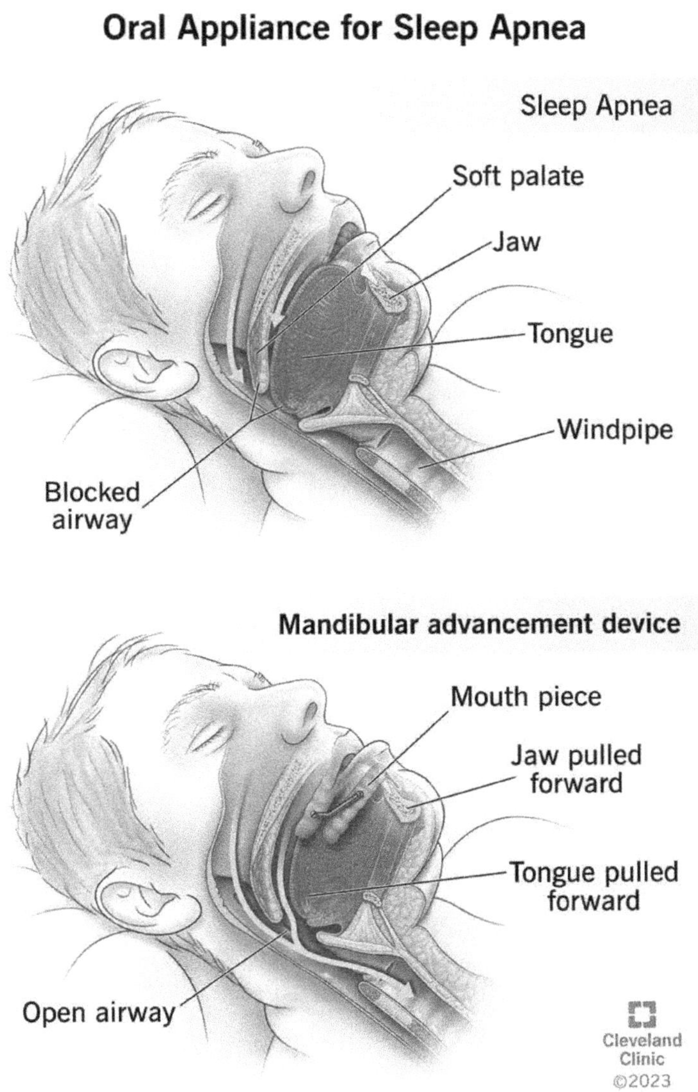

Fig 11: Oral appliances

Tongue-stabilizing devices

Another name for tongue-stabilizing devices (TSDs) is tongue-retaining devices. They use suction to force your tongue forward in order to treat OSA

The gadget's suction bulb keeps your tongue in place while you're asleep. A TSD's tip remains outside of your mouth. Similar to MADs, TSDs cause the base of your tongue to move forward, opening your airway. 100.

Although TSDs are less common than MADs, they might be a choice for OSA sufferers who wish to test an oral appliance but are unable to use MADs. For instance, a TSD may be used in place of a MAD by those whose teeth are too weak. Additionally, these can be purchased over-the-counter.

The best oral device for treating sleep apnea

The best oral appliances are manufactured specifically to fit your mouth. Oral appliances, such as "boil and bite" types that take an impression of your teeth, are available without a prescription. Although studies indicates that custom-made oral appliances provide the best results for OSA, these types may still be beneficial.[100]

How does oral appliance therapy work to treat obstructive sleep apnea?

By pulling the base of the tongue forward, oral appliances increase the amount of space in the back of the throat. Certain varieties grab the tongue and drag it forward. While the tongue stays still, most drag the lower jaw forward.

Before going to bed, the patient puts the device on, wears it all night, and takes it off when they wake up.

Benefits of oral appliance therapy for obstructive sleep apnea (OSA)

- It can alleviate OSA symptoms, such as difficulty concentrating and daytime tiredness.
- Some people find that their sleep is deeper and less disturbed.
- Reduction or elimination of snoring is possible.
- For those who are unable to utilize a CPAP, it provides an alternative.
- Traveling with it is a breeze.

Side effects of oral appliance therapy for OSA Short-term side effects include:

- When the device is in your mouth, you will spit more.
- Pain in the jaw, teeth, and temporomandibular joint (TMJ).
- The mouth is parched
- inflammation of the gums.

When an appliance is fitted correctly, long-term negative effects are rare. When problems arise, they consist of:

- Your bite has changed.
- Teeth can move or come loose.
- Your TMJ or jaw muscles may change.

Multidisciplinary approach in management of OSA [101] Role of orthodontist

- Orthodontists are essential in managing OSA, mostly through the following interventions: -OSA can be effectively treated with surgical-orthodontic maxillomandibular advancement, particularly in individuals with skeletal disharmonies. It improves airway capacity and decreases collapsibility, but for best results, careful patient selection and accurate phenotyping are necessary.
- One effective non-surgical therapy option for OSA is mandibular advancement appliances. By moving the jaw forward, they increase airway patency and are linked to significant symptom relief and excellent patient compliance. In both adults and children with OSA and maxillary constriction, Rapid Maxillary Expansion has demonstrated favorable results.

- Although its effectiveness varies, it raises nasal and oropharyngeal airway volumes. More research is required to determine which endotypes and phenotypes respond best to this treatment.

Role of otolaryngologist

ENT conditions that affect the pathophysiology of OSA, including as tonsillar hypertrophy, allergic rhinitis, inferior turbinate hypertrophy, deviated nasal septum, and high Mallampati score, were more prevalent in OSA patients than in simple snorers. its mode of therapy.

These ENT factors contribute to a less collapsible upper airway during sleep because they are reasonably easy to identify and can be corrected with safe, straightforward medicinal and/or surgical procedures. Therefore, it will be beneficial for all individuals with sleep disordered breathing to have an ENT evaluation. As a result, otolaryngologists are essential to the treatment of pediatric OSA.

Role of Pulmonologist

CPAP therapy is considered the most effective treatment for people with moderate or severe OSA. A patient using CPAP must cover their airway while they sleep using an interface, such as an oronasal or nasal mask. In order to prevent the patient's upper airway from collapsing, compressed room air is created by connecting the mask via a tube to a bedside device that is often powered by the mains. But each time the patients go to sleep, the treatment needs to be given. Proper adherence to CPAP therapy removes intermittent hypoxia, sleep fragmentation, and nocturnal apneas and hypopneas for most patients undergoing treatment. By lowering EDS and other effects that would have been brought on by unmanaged OSA, like hypertension, it also greatly enhances the patient's quality of life.[98].

Role of Maxillofacial surgeon

In an effort to widen their retro lingual and retropalatal airways, patients with obstruction in either the hypopharynx or the tongue base are given maxillomandibular advancement (MMA), which involves advancing both the maxilla and the mandible. The maxillofacial surgeon is among the several medical professionals who must approve this invasive treatment.

ROLE OF PEDODONTIST IN MANAGEMENT OF PAEDIATRIC OSA

Children frequently suffer from pediatric obstructive sleep apnea, which is linked to a number of health issues.ThepossibilitythatPOSAwouldgountreatedorbedelayedinmanychildrenduetothelackofavailable resources is equally concerning. lab for pediatric polysomnography 97. If POSA is not treated, there are a number of potentially detrimental outcomes, such as behavioral or attention issues, poor academic performance, cardiovascular disease, and growth and nutritional issues ranging from obesity to failure to thrive. It is recommended that all dentists learn about the screening methods, diagnosis, and treatment of POSA due to its high prevalence in youngsters.

According to the current literature, pedodontists should provide children with modern oral health care that includes: (1) education on the epidemiology, pathophysiology, and treatment considerations of children with POSA (only doctors can diagnose POSA); (2) routine history, questionnaires, and clinical screening, along with appropriate referrals to the medical team members; (3) integration with the medical team in addressing POSA; and (4) obtaining the higher education required to fabricate and deliver oral appliances only after a thorough orthodontic examination for a comprehensive multidisciplinary approach.One hundred. Therefore, it is advised that the screening and treatment of children with POSA be included in the core curricula of all dental schools and postgraduate dental training programs. To prevent negative consequences when treating POSA, only treating dentists who have received further training in this field should be employed for this multidisciplinary position.

Furthermore, more significant clinical research is required to confirm dental treatment strategies for this particular age range because POSA often affects children between the ages of 2 and 7 and there is a lack of data regarding dental treatment approaches for this age group. Pedodontists can significantly improve the care of children with POSA and become important contributors to the science of POSA by carefully collaborating with physicians and other healthcare professionals. This will have a positive impact on the health and quality of life of their pediatric patients. [101].

Complications of Pediatric OSA

In pediatric practice, obstructive apnea, particularly OSA, is a prevalent issue. Craniofacial abnormalities may be the most frequent cause of OSA in young newborns. Failure to thrive, metabolic alkalosis, and potentially fatal respiratory distress are among the complications 103. Adenoidal and tonsillar hypertrophy are more frequently the cause of upper airway obstruction in children older than two. Adult respiratory distress syndrome, cor pulmonale, and growth failure consequences were discussed. Children and newborns with obstructive sleep apnea may have serious problems. These issues may be fatal, impede growth and development, or result in mild long-term learning difficulties.

Pediatric OSA can have major morbidities and long-term problems if treatment is not received. At a young age, pulmonary hypertension, right heart failure, and increased pulmonary vasoconstriction can result from prolonged hypoxia 102. Undiagnosed and untreated pediatric OSA is linked to cognitive dysfunction, learning impairment, and poor academic performance. Furthermore, failure to thrive in younger populations may be linked to greater respiratory effort.

However, like with any surgical procedure, it must be acknowledged that it is not harmless and should be carefully evaluated. There are specific surgical risks and consequences that come with using A&T on a patient. [103].

Sadly, even though they are uncommon in children, tonsillectomy can have negative side effects. Localized discomfort, reduced oral intake, and dehydration during the acute post-surgical period are the most prevalent. Bleeding, secondary infection, respiratory compromise, velopharyngeal insufficiency, and subglottic stenosis are more worrisome A&T consequences. There is always a chance of bronchospasm or laryngospasm, just like with any surgery requiring airway control 104. A higher risk of post-surgical problems is predicted by a higher degree of OSA severity, and patients with more severe OSA may need more time in the PACU or inpatient ward following surgery.[67]

Some congenital and medical conditions associated with OSA

Obstructive sleep apnea in children with Downs syndrome

Obstructive sleep apnea (OSA) is a sleep-related disorder that can affect both adults and children. Depending on the disease's severity and phenotype, OSA can have both immediate and long-term effects. It is characterized by recurrent partial or total upper airway blockage during sleep, which causes sporadic bouts of hypoxia and sleep fragmentation 105. Excessive daily sleepiness, fatigue, behavioral and mental issues, low quality of life, and poor academic performance are some signs of OSA in children. Cardiovascular consequences, such as pulmonary hypertension, diminished autonomic reflexes, and blood pressure dysregulation, are widely recognized.

The most prevalent genetic chromosomal disease in people is Down syndrome (DS). In 95% of cases, nondisjunction during cell division results in three copies of chromosome 21 in each embryonic cell. In roughly 4% of cases, a section of chromosome 21 may be translocated onto another chromosome during division. Less than 1% of persons have mosaicism, a condition in which a few body cells have three copies of chromosome 21. Classic dysmorphic features include a brachycephalic head, epicanthal folds, upward-slanting palpebral fissures, a flat nasal bridge, a small mouth and ears, a short neck with an additional fat pad, a single palmar crease, a significant space between the first and second toes, and hypotonia. The majority of people with Down syndrome (DS) have a moderate level of cognitive impairment, with an intelligence quotient (IQ) between 35 and 50.

Congenital heart disease, hearing and visual issues, thyroid disorders, and OSA are common medical conditions linked to DS.[99]

Diabetes and Sleep Health: How circadian rhythm, sleep length, and subjective sleep affect diabetes[97]

Obstructive sleep apnea (OSA) is a respiratory disorder characterized by partial or total obstruction of the upper airway during sleep, resulting in repeated episodes of reflexive awakenings (apneas and hypopneas) to get enough oxygen and air. Episodes of apnea and hypopnea can cause physiological stress and oxygen desaturation, jeopardizing vital homeostatic physiological functions.

The cardiometabolic system, where untreated OSA causes metabolic problems, is compromised by recurrent cycles of apnea and hypopnea. Research has shown that sleep fragmentation, shorter sleep duration, and occasional hypoxia (oxygen loss from apnea and hypopnea) have negative impacts on glucose metabolism. Clinicians must address the significant probability of concomitant OSA risk and type 2 diabetes among their patients in light of the aforementioned research.

Sleep apnea and cardiometabolic disease

The most prevalent type of respiratory disturbance during sleep is obstructive sleep apnea (OSA). The recurring collapse of the upper airway's soft tissues, which causes a partial or total halt of airflow, is the hallmark of OSA. Crucially, OSA differs from central sleep apnea in that OSA sufferers keep trying to breathe during the apnea. Over the past 20 years, as sleep apnea diagnoses have increased, treatment options have changed, and our understanding of how sleep apnea contributes to cardiovascular disease has improved, the mechanisms underlying obstructive sleep apnea have been the focus of extensive research.[105].

The oro- and nasopharyngeal spaces, which define the upper airways, are adaptable, multipurpose structures that support respiration, phonation, mastication, deglutition of solids and liquids, and secretion clearance. The upper airway is supported by a complex network of muscles rather than the stiff cartilaginous support system found in the first few generations of lower airways. Swallowing and phonation require both full and partial airway closure. However, when closure happens repeatedly while you're asleep, this ability becomes pathological. Patients with obstructive sleep apnea experience respiratory episodes frequently enough to have clinical effects, despite disagreements over the threshold for normal versus abnormal.[105].

Conclusion

A strong index of suspicion and inquiry are necessary to assess the severity and current comorbidities of pediatric sleep apnea, a commonly overlooked condition. Pediatricians and respiratory doctors need to be made more aware in order to help them identify and act quickly. When surgery is not a possibility, positive airway pressure and medication therapy are good substitutes. In severe situations, adenotonsillectomy is still the major surgical procedure. Restoring functional activities in sleep-disordered breathing requires close monitoring and multidisciplinary intervention.

References

1. Sateia MJ. International classification of sleep disorders-third edition: highlights and modifications. Chest. 2014 Nov;146(5):1387-1394.
2. Tauman R, Gozal D. Obstructive sleep apnea syndrome in children. Expert Review of Respiratory Medicine 2011;5(3):425–40.
3. Guilleminault C, Eldridge FL, Simmons FB, Dement WC. Sleep apnea in eight children. Pediatrics 1976;58(1):23–30.
4. Busby KA, Mercier L, Pivik RT. Ontogenetic variations in auditory arousal threshold during sleep. Psychophysiology 1994;31(2):182–8.
5. Löfstrand-Tideström B, Thilander B, Ahlqvist-Rastad J, Jakobsson O, Hultcrantz E. Breathing obstruction in relation to craniofacial and dental arch morphology in 4- yearold children. The European Journal of Orthodontics 1999;21(4):323–32.
6. Goh DY, Galster P, Marcus CL. Sleep architecture and respiratory disturbances in children withobstructive sleep apnea. Am. J. Respir. Crit. Care Med. 2000;162(2 Pt 1):682–6.
7. Goldbart AD, Goldman JL, Veling MC, Gozal D. Leukotriene modifier therapy for mild sleep-disordered breathing in children. Am. J. Respir. Crit. Care Med. 2005;172(3):364–70.
8. American Academy of Sleep Medicine. International Classification of Sleep Disorders – ThirdEdition (ICSD-3). Amer Academy of Sleep Medicine; 2014.
9. Bickelmann AG, Burwell CS, Robin ED, Whaley RD. Extreme obesity associated with alveolar hypoventilation: a Pickwickian syndrome. Am J Med. 1956 Nov; 21(5):811- 818.
10. Jordan AS, McSharry DG, Malhotra A. Adult obstructive sleep apnoea. Lancet. 2014 Feb;383(9918):736–747.
11. Watson NF, Badr MS, Belenky G, et al. Joint consensus statement of the American Academy of Sleep Medicine and Sleep Research Society on the recommended amount of sleep for a healthy adult: methodology and discussion. J Clin Sleep Med. 2015;11(8):931–952.
12. Luyster FS, Strollo PJ, Zee PC, Walsh JK; Boards of Directors of the American Academy of Sleep Medicine and the Sleep Research Society. Sleep: a health imperative. Sleep. 2012;35(6):727–734.
13. Ohayon M, Wickwire EM, Hirshkowitz M, et al. National Sleep Foundation's sleep quality recommendations: first report. Sleep Health. 2017;3(1):6–19.

14. Watson NF, Badr MS, Belenky G, et al. Recommended amount of sleep for a healthy adult: a joint consensus statement of the American Academy of Sleep Medicine and Sleep Research Society. J Clin Sleep Med. 2015;11(6):591–592.

15. Loomis AL, Harvey EN, Hobart GA. Cerebral states during sleep as studied by human brainpotentials. Journal of Experimental Psychology. 1937;21(2):127–144.

16. Zepelin H, Siegel JM, Tobler I. Mammalian sleep. In: Kryger MH, Roth T, Dement WC, editors. Principles and Practice of Sleep Medicine. 4th ed. Philadelphia: Elsevier/Saunders;2005. pp. 91–100.

17. Carskadon M, Dement W. Normal human sleep: An overview. In: Kryger MH, Roth T, Dement WC, editors. Principles and Practice of Sleep Medicine. 4th ed. Philadelphia: Elsevier Saunders;2005. pp. 13–23.

18. Gillette M, Abbott S. Sleep Research Society. SRS Basics of Sleep Guide. Westchester, IL: Sleep Research Society; 2005. Fundamentals of the circadian system; pp. 131–138.

19. Somers V, Dyken M, Mark A, Abboud F. Sympathetic-nerve activity during sleep in normal subjects. New England Journal of Medicine. 1993;328(5):303–307.

20. Dunlap JC, Loros JJ, DeCoursey PJ. Chronobiology: Biological Timekeeping. Sunderland, MA: Sinauer Associates; 2004.

21. Bunning E. The Physiological Clock. Berlin, Germany: Springer-Verlag; 1964.

22. Vitaterna M, Pinto L, Turek F. Molecular genetic basis for mammalian circadian rhythms. In: Kryger MH, Roth T, Dement WC, editors. Principles and Practice of Sleep Medicine. 4th ed. Philadelphia: Elsevier/Saunders; 2005. pp. 363–374.

23. Sankri-Tarbichi AG. Obstructive sleep apnea-hypopnea syndrome: Etiology and diagnosis. Avicenna J Med. 2012 Jan;2(1):3-8.

24. Mehrtash M, Bakker JP, Ayas N. Predictors of Continuous Positive Airway Pressure Adherence in Patients with Obstructive Sleep Apnea. Lung. 2019 Apr;197(2):115- 121.

25. Yeghiazarians Y, Jneid H, Tietjens JR, Redline S, Brown DL, El-Sherif N, Mehra R, Bozkurt B, Ndumele CE, Somers VK. Obstructive Sleep Apnea and Cardiovascular Disease: A Scientific Statement From the American Heart Association. Circulation. 2021 Jul 20;144(3):e56-e67.

26. Isono S, Remmers JE, Tanaka A, Sho Y, Sato J, Nishino T. Anatomy of pharynx in patients with obstructive sleep apnea and in normal subjects. J Appl Physiol (1985). 1997 Apr;82(4):1319-26.

27. Tufik S, Santos-Silva R, Taddei JA, Bittencourt LR. Obstructive sleep apnea syndrome in the Sao Paulo Epidemiologic Sleep Study. Sleep Med. 2010 May; 11(5):441-6.

28. Bixler EO, Vgontzas AN, Ten Have T, Tyson K, Kales A. Effects of age on sleep apnea in men: I. Prevalence and severity. Am J Respir Crit Care Med. 1998 Jan;157(1):144-8.

29. Wenzel SE. Asthma phenotypes: the evolution from clinical to molecular approaches. Nat Med. 2012;18(5):716–25.

30. Zinchuk AV, Gentry MJ, Concato J, Yaggi HK. Phenotypes in obstructive sleep apnea: A definition, examples and evolution of approaches. Sleep Med Rev. 2017 Oct;35:113-123.

31. Brietzke SE, Katz ES, Roberson DW. Can history and physical examination reliably diagnose pediatric obstructive sleep apnea/hypopnea syndrome? A systematic review of the literature. Otolaryngol Head Neck Surg2004;131:827-32.

32. Luz Alonso-Álvarez M., Canet T., Cubell-Alarco M., Estivill E., Fernández-Julián E., Gozal D., Jurado-Luque M.J., Lluch-Roselló M.A., Martínez-Pérez F., Merino- Andreu M., et al. Documento de consenso del síndrome de apneas- hipopneasduranteelsueñoenniños (versióncompleta) Arch. Bronconeumol. 2011;47:2–18.

33. Kaditis A.G., Alonso Alvarez M.L., Boudewyns A., Alexopoulos E.I., Ersu R., Joosten K., Larramona H., Miano S., Narang I., Trang H., et al. Obstructive Sleep

34. Disordered Breathing in 2- to 18-Year-Old Children: Diagnosis and Management. Eur. Respir. J. 2016;47:69–94.

35. Marcus C.L., Brooks L.J., Ward S.D., Draper K.A., Gozal D., Halbower A.C., Jones J., Lehmann C., Schechter M.S., Sheldon S., et al. Diagnosis and Management of Childhood Obstructive Sleep Apnea Syndrome. Pediatrics. 2012;130:e714–e755.

36. Dayyat E, Kheirandish-Gozal L, Gozal D. Childhood obstructive sleep apnea: one or two distinct disease entities? Clin Sleep Med 2007;42:374–379.

37. Lavie P. Nothing new under the moon. Historical accounts of sleep apnea syndrome. Arch Intern Med 1984;144:2025–2028

38. Jung R, Kuhlo W. Neurophysiological studies of abnormal night sleep and the Pickwickian syndrome. Prog Brain Res 1965;18:140–159.

39. Young T, Palta M, Dempsey J, Skatrud J, Weber S, Badr S. The occurrence of sleepdisordered breathing among middle-aged adults. N Engl J Med 1993;328:1230–1235.

40. Stradling JR, Crosby JH. Predictors and prevalence of obstructive sleep apnoea and snoring in 1001 middle aged men. Thorax 1991;46:85–90.

41. Jennum P, Sjøl A. Epidemiology of snoring and obstructive sleep apnoea in a Danish population, age 30–60. J Sleep Res 1992;1:240–244.

42. Durán J, Esnaola S, Rubio R, Iztueta A. Obstructive sleep apnea–hypopnea and related clinical features in a population-based sample of subjects aged 30 to 70 yr. Am J Respir Crit Care Med 2001;163:685–689.

43. White DP. Pathogenesis of obstructive and central sleep apnea. Am J Respir Crit Care Med 2005;172: 1363–1370

44. Eckert DJ, Malhotra A. Pathophysiology of adult obstructive sleep apnea. Proc Am Thorac Soc. 2008 Feb 15;5(2):144-53.

45. Schwab RJ, Gupta KB, Gefter WB, Metzger LJ, Hoffman EA, Pack AI. Upper airway and soft tissue anatomy in normal subjects and patients with sleep-disordered breathing: significance of the lateral pharyngeal walls. Am J Respir Crit Care Med 1995;152: 1673–1689.

46. Mezzanotte WS, Tangel DJ, White DP. Waking genioglossal electromyogram in sleep apnea patients versus normal controls (a neuromuscular compensatory mechanism). J Clin Invest 1992;89: 1571–1579.

47. Mezzanotte WS, Tangel DJ, White DP. Influence of sleep onset on upper-airway muscle activity in apnea patients versus normal controls. Am J Respir Crit Care Med 1996;153: 1880–1887.

48. Trinder J, Whitworth F, Kay A, Wilkin P. Respiratory instability during sleep onset. J Appl Physiol 1992;73: 2462–2469.

49. Basner RC, Ringler J, Schwartzstein RM, Weinberger SE, Weiss JW. Phasic electromyographic activity of the genioglossus increases in normals during slow- wave sleep. Respir Physiol 1991;83: 189–200.

50. Pillar G, Fogel RB, Malhotra A, Beauregard J, Edwards JK, Shea SA, White DP. Genioglossal inspiratory activation: central respiratory vs mechanoreceptive influences. Respir Physiol 2001;127: 23–38.

51. Horner RL, Innes JA, Murphy K, Guz A. Evidence for reflex upper airway dilator muscle activation by sudden negative airway pressure in man. J Physiol 1991;436: 15–29

52. Horner RL, Innes JA, Morrell MJ, Shea SA, Guz A. The effect of sleep on reflex genioglossus muscle activation by stimuli of negative airway pressure in humans. J Physiol 1994;476: 141–151.

53. Jordan AS, Wellman A, Heinzer RC, Lo YL, Schory K, Dover L, Gautam S, Malhotra A, White DP. Mechanisms used to restore ventilation after partial upper airway collapse during sleep in humans. Thorax 2007;62: 861–867.

54. Phillipson EA, Sullivan CE. Arousal: the forgotten response to respiratory stimuli. Am Rev Respir Dis 1978;118: 807–809.

55. Nigro CA, Rhodius EE. Variation in the duration of arousal in obstructive sleep apnea. Med Sci Monit 2005;11:CR188–CR192

56. Younes M. Role of arousals in the pathogenesis of obstructive sleep apnea. Am J Respir Crit Care Med 2004;169: 623–633.

57. Khoo MC, Kronauer RE, Strohl KP, Slutsky AS. Factors inducing periodic breathing in humans: a general model. J Appl Physiol 1982;53: 644–659.

58. Stanchina ML, Ellison K, Malhotra A, Anderson M, Kirk M, Benser ME, Tosi C, Carlisle C, Millman RP, Buxton A. The impact of cardiac resynchronization therapy on obstructive sleep apnea in heart failure patients: a pilot study. Chest 2007;132: 433–439.

59. Luzzi V, Altieri F, Guaragna M, Pirro V, Marasca B, Cotticelli L, Mazur M, Di Carlo G, Di Giacomo P, Di Paolo C, Brunori M, Ierardo G, Piperno G, Magliulo G, Pace A, Iannella G, Palange P, Martini A, Pietrafesa E, Polimeni A. Friedman Tongue Position and the Anthropometric Parameters in Adult Patients with Obstructive Sleep Apnea: An Observational Study. Int J Environ Res Public Health. 2023 Feb 13;20(4):3255.

60. Ravesloot MJL, Van Maanen J, Hilgevoord A, Van Wagensveld B, De Vries N. Obstructive sleep apnea is underrecognized and underdiagnosed in patients undergoing bariatric surger y. European Archives of Oto-Rhino-Laryngology. 2012;269(7):1865–71.

61. Shelton KE, Woodson H, Gay S, Suratt PM. Pharyngeal fat in obstructive sleep apnea. Am Rev Respir Dis. 1993;148(2):462–466.

62. Naimark A, Cherniack RM. Compliance of the respiratory system and its components in health and obesity. J Appl Physiol. 1960;15: 377–382.

63. Malhotra A, White DP. Obstructive sleep apnoea. Lancet. 2002;360(9328):237–245.

64. Phillips BG, Hisel TM, Kato M, et al. Recent weight gain in patients with newly diagnosed obstructive sleep apnea. J Hypertens. 1999;17(9):1297–1300.

65. Spiegel K, Tasali E, Penev P, Van Cauter E. Brief communication: sleep curtailment in healthy young men is associated with decreased leptin levels, elevated ghrelin levels, and increased hunger and appetite. Ann Intern Med. 2004;141(11):846–850.

66. Vgontzas AN, Papanicolaou DA, Bixler EO, et al. Sleep apnea and daytime sleepiness and fatigue: relation to visceral obesity, insulin resistance, and hypercytokinemia. J Clin Endocrinol Metab. 2000;85(3):1151–1158.

67. Chin K, Shimizu K, Nakamura T, et al. Changes in intra-abdominal visceral fat and serum leptin levels in patients with obstructive sleep apnea syndrome following nasal continuous positive airway pressure therapy. Circulation. 1999;100(7):706– 712.

68. Patel SR, Larkin EK, Redline S. Shared genetic basis for obstructive sleep apnea and adiposity measures. Int J Obes (Lond) 2008;32(5):795–800.

69. Popko K, Gorska E, Wasik M, et al. Frequency of distribution of leptin gene polymorphism in obstructive sleep apnea patients. J PhysiolPharmacol. 2007;58(Pt. 2) Suppl 5:551–561.

70. Schwengel DA, Dalesio NM, Stierer TL. Pediatric bstructive sleep apnea. Anesthesiol Clin. 2014 Mar;32(1):237-61

71. Celestin J, Lockey RF. Pediatric Sleep Apnea Syndrome: An Update. J Allergy Clin Immunol Pract. 2016 Sep-Oct;4(5):852-61.

72. Rosen D. Management of obstructive sleep apnea associated with Down syndrome and other craniofacial dysmorphologies. Curr OpinPulm Med. 2011 Nov;17(6):431- 6.

73. Garg RK, Afifi AM, Garland CB, Sanchez R, Mount DL. Pediatric Obstructive Sleep Apnea: Consensus, Controversy, and Craniofacial Considerations. Plast Reconstr Surg. 2017 Nov;140(5):987-997.

74. Medicine AAoS. International classification of sleep disorders— third edition (ICSD-3) Darien, Illinois: 2014.

75. AASM. Manual for the Scoring of Sleep and Associated Events, Version 2.3. 2016 Apr 1.

76. Karimi M, Hedner J, Häbel H, Nerman O, Grote L. Sleep apnea related risk of motor vehicle accidents is reduced by continuous positive air way pressure: Swedish traffic accident registry data. Sleep. 2015;38(3):341.

77. Mallampati SR, Gatt SP, Gugino LD, Desai SP, Waraksa B, Freiberger D, Liu PL. A clinical sign to predict difficult tracheal intubation: a prospective study. Can Anaesth Soc J. 1985 Jul;32(4):429-34.

78. Chung F, Abdullah HR, Liao P. STOP-Bang Questionnaire: A practical approach to screen for obstructive sleep apnea. CHEST Journal. 2016;149(3):631–8.

79. Kasai T, Floras JS, Bradley TD. Sleep apnea and cardiovascular disease: a bidirectional relationship. Circulation 2012;126: 1495-510.

80. Tilkian AG, Guilleminault C, Schroeder JS, et al. Hemodynamics in sleep-induced apnea. Studies during wakefulness and sleep. Ann Intern Med 1976;85: 714-9.

81. Tilkian AG, Guilleminault C, Schroeder JS, et al. Sleep-induced apnea syndrome. Prevalence of cardiac arrhythmias and their reversal after tracheostomy. Am J Med 1977;63: 348-58.

82. Javaheri S. Sleep disorders in systolic heart failure: a prospective study of 100 male patients. The final report. Int J Cardiol 2006;106: 21-8.

83. Simonneau G, Gatzoulis MA, Adatia I, et al. Updated clinical classification of pulmonary hypertension. J Am Coll Cardiol 2013;62: D34-41.

84. Bonsignore MR, Borel AL, Machan E, et al. Sleep apnoea and metabolic dysfunction. Eur Respir Rev 2013;22: 353-64.

85. Kheirandish-Gozal L, Bandla HP, Gozal D. Montelukast for Children with Obstructive Sleep Apnea: Results of a Double-Blind, Randomized, Placebo- Controlled Trial. Ann Am Thorac Soc. 2016 Oct;13(10):1736-1741.

86. Cielo CM, Gungor A. Treatment Options for Pediatric Obstructive Sleep Apnea. Curr ProblPediatrAdolesc Health Care. 2016 Jan;46(1):27-33.

87. Camacho M, Certal V, Abdullatif J, Zaghi S, Ruoff CM, Capasso R, Kushida CA. Myofunctional Therapy to Treat Obstructive Sleep Apnea: A Systematic Review and Meta-analysis. Sleep. 2015 May 01;38(5):669-75.

88. Hawkins S, Huston S, Campbell K, Halbower A. High- Flow, heated, humidified air via nasal cannula treats CPAP- intolerant children with obstructive sleep apnea. J Clin Sleep Med. 2017;13: 981- 989.

89. Wellman A, Malhotra A, Jordan AS, Stevenson KE, Gautam S, White DP. Effect of oxygen in obstructive sleep apnea: role of loop gain. Respir PhysiolNeurobiol. 2008;162: 144- 151.

90. Yu JL, Afolabi-Brown O. Updates on management of pediatric obstructive sleep apnea. PediatrInvestig. 2019 Dec 21;3(4):228-235.

91. Schechter M.S. Section on Pediatric Pulmonology, Subcommittee on Obstructive Sleep Apnea Syndrome. Technical report: Diagnosis and management of childhood obstructive sleep apnea syndrome. Pediatrics. 2002;109: e69.

92. Tagaya M., Nakata S., Yasuma F., Mitchell R.B., Sasaki F., Miyazaki S., Morinaga M., Otake H., Teranishi M., Nakashima T. Children with severe or moderate obstructive sleep apnoeasyndrome show a high incidence of persistence afteradenotonsillectomy. Acta Otolaryngol. 2012;132: 1208–1214.

93. Cielo CM, Duffy KA, Taylor JA, Marcus CL, Kalish JM. Obstructive Sleep Apnea in Children With Beckwith- Wiedemann Syndrome. J Clin Sleep Med. 2019;15: 375381.

94. Thorne MC, Garetz SL. Laryngomalacia: review and summary of current clinical practice in 2015. Paediatr Respir Rev. 2016;17: 3- 8.

95. Guilleminault C, Simmons FB, Motta J, Cummiskey J, Rosekind M, Schroeder JS, et al.Obstructive sleep apnea syndrome and tracheostomy. Long- term follow- up experience. Arch Intern Med. 1981;141: 985- 988.

96. Rizzi CJ, Amin JD, Isaiah A, Valdez TA, Jeyakumar A, Smart SE, et al. Tracheostomy for severe pediatric obstructive sleep apnea : Indications a nd out comes. Otolaryngol Head Neck Surg. 2017;157: 309-313.

97. Croft CB, Pringle M. Sleep nasendoscopy: a technique of assessment in snoring and obstructive sleep apnoea. Clin Otolaryngol Allied Sci. 1991;16: 504- 509.

98. Donnelly LF, Casper KA, Chen B, Koch BL. Defining normal upper airway motion in asymptomatic children during sleep by means of cine MR techniques. Radiology. 2002;223: 176- 180.

99. O'Connor E.A., Evans C.V., Burda B.U., Walsh E.S., Eder M., Lozano P. Screening for Obesity and Intervention for Weight Management in Children and Adolescents: Evidence Report and Systematic Review for the US Preventive Services Task Force. JAMA. 2017;317: 2427–2444.

100. Hady KK, Okorie CUA. Positive Airway Pressure Therapy for Pediatric Obstructive Sleep Apnea. Children (Basel). 2021 Oct 29;8(11):979.

101. Croft C.B., Thomson H.G., Samuels M.P., Southall D.P. Endoscopic evaluation and treatment of sleep-associated upper airway obstruction in infants and young children. Clin. Otolaryngol. Allied Sci. 1990;15: 209–216.

102. Rosen C.L. Clinical features of obstructive sleep apnea hypoventilation syndrome in otherwise healthy children. Pediatr. Pulmonol. 1999;27: 403–409.

103. Feng X, Chen Y, Hellén-Halme K, Cai W, Shi XQ. The effect of rapid maxillary expansion on the upper airway's aerodynamic characteristics. BMC Oral Health. 2021 Mar 17;21(1):123.

104. Randerath WJ, Verbraecken J, Andreas S, Bettega G, Boudewyns A, Hamans E, et al. Non-CPAP therapies in obstructive sleep apnoea. Eur Respir J. (2011) 37:1000– 28.

105. Carvalho FR, Lentini-Oliveira DA, Prado LB, Prado GF, Carvalho LB. Oral appliances and functional orthopaedic appliances for obstructive sleep apnoea in children. Cochrane Database Syst Rev. 2016 Oct 5;10(10)

106. Arachchige MA, Steier J. Beyond Usual Care: A Multidisciplinary Approach Towards the Treatment of Obstructive Sleep Apnoea. Front Cardiovasc Med. 2022 Jan 5;8: 747495.

107. Grout RW, Cunniff C, Parisi MA, Ralston SJ, Scott JA, Shapira SK, Spire P. Health Supervision for Children and Adolescents With Down Syndrome. Pediatrics. 2022 May 1;149(5).

www.ingramcontent.com/pod-product-compliance
Lightning Source LLC
LaVergne TN
LVHW070911210926
848482LV00017B/1049